Statistical Analysis of Spatial Point Patterns

Second Edition

Peter J Diggle
Professor of Statistics, Lancaster University
Adjunct Professor of Biostatistics, John Hopkins University

A member of the Hodder Headline Group
LONDON
Distributed in the United States of America by
Oxford University Press Inc., New York

First published in Great Britain in 1983
This edition published in 2003 by
Arnold, a member of the Hodder Headline Group,
338 Euston Road, London NW1 3BH

http://www.arnoldpublishers.com

Distributed in the United States of America by
Oxford University Press Inc.,
198 Madison Avenue, New York, NY10016

© 2003 Peter J Diggle

All rights reserved. No part of this publication may be reproduced or
transmitted in any form or by any means, electronically or mechanically,
including photocopying, recording or any information storage or retrieval
system, without either prior permission in writing from the publisher or a
licence permitting restricted copying. In the United Kingdom such licences
are issued by the Copyright Licensing Agency: 90 Tottenham Court Road,
London W1T 4LP.

The advice and information in this book are believed to be true and
accurate at the date of going to press, but neither the author[s] nor the publisher
can accept any legal responsibility or liability for any errors or omissions.

British Library Cataloguing in Publication Data
A catalogue record for this book is available from the British Library

Library of Congress Cataloging-in-Publication Data
A catalog record for this book is available from the Library of Congress

ISBN 0 340 74070 1 (hb)

1 2 3 4 5 6 7 8 9 10

Production Controller: Martin Kerans
Cover Design: Terry Griffiths

Typeset in 10/11 pt Times by Charon Tec Pvt. Ltd, Chennai, India
Printed and bound in Great Britain by MPG Books, Bodmin, Cornwall

> What do you think about this book? Or any other Arnold title?
> Please send your comments to feedback.arnold@hodder.co.uk

Contents

Preface   vii

1. Introduction   1
    1.1 Spatial point patterns   1
    1.2 Sampling   3
    1.3 Edge effects   5
    1.4 Complete spatial randomness   6
    1.5 Objectives of statistical analysis   7
    1.6 The Dirichlet tessellation   8
    1.7 Monte Carlo tests   9
    1.8 Software   10

2. Preliminary testing   12
    2.1 Tests of complete spatial randomness   12
    2.2 Inter-event distances   13
       2.2.1 Analysis of Japanese black pine saplings   14
       2.2.2 Analysis of redwood seedlings   14
       2.2.3 Analysis of biological cells   16
       2.2.4 Small distances   16
    2.3 Nearest neighbour distances   17
       2.3.1 Analysis of Japanese black pine saplings   19
       2.3.2 Analysis of redwood seedlings   19
       2.3.3 Analysis of biological cells   19
    2.4 Point-to-nearest-event distances   21
       2.4.1 Analysis of Japanese black pine saplings   22
       2.4.2 Analysis of redwood seedlings   22
       2.4.3 Analysis of biological cells   22
    2.5 Quadrat counts   23
       2.5.1 Analysis of Japanese black pine saplings   24
       2.5.2 Analysis of redwood seedlings   24
       2.5.3 Analysis of biological cells   25
    2.6 Scales of pattern   25
       2.6.1 Analysis of Lansing Woods data   26
       2.6.2 Scales of dependence   27
    2.7 Recommendations   28

3. Statistical methods for sparsely sampled patterns — 30
- 3.1 General remarks — 30
- 3.2 Quadrat counts — 31
  - 3.2.1 Tests of CSR — 31
  - 3.2.2 Estimators of intensity — 32
  - 3.2.3 Analysis of Lansing Woods data — 32
- 3.3 Distance methods — 33
  - 3.3.1 Distribution theory under CSR — 33
  - 3.3.2 Tests of CSR — 35
  - 3.3.3 Estimators of intensity — 39
  - 3.3.4 Analysis of Lansing Woods data — 40
- 3.4 Tests of independence — 40
- 3.5 Recommendations — 41

4. Spatial point processes — 42
- 4.1 Processes and summary descriptions — 42
- 4.2 Second-order properties — 43
  - 4.2.1 Univariate processes — 43
  - 4.2.2 Extension to multivariate processes — 45
- 4.3 Higher-order moments and nearest neighbour distributions — 46
- 4.4 The homogeneous Poisson process — 47
- 4.5 Independence and random labelling — 48
- 4.6 Estimation of second-order properties — 49
  - 4.6.1 Univariate processes — 49
  - 4.6.2 Inhomogeneous processes — 55
  - 4.6.3 Multivariate processes — 55
  - 4.6.4 Examples — 56
- 4.7 Displaced amacrine cells in the retina of a rabbit — 58
- 4.8 Estimation of nearest neighbour distributions — 60
  - 4.8.1 Examples — 61
- 4.9 Concluding remarks — 62

5. Models — 63
- 5.1 Introduction — 63
- 5.2 Contagious distributions — 63
- 5.3 Poisson cluster processes — 64
- 5.4 Inhomogeneous Poisson processes — 67
- 5.5 Cox processes — 68
- 5.6 Simple inhibition processes — 72
- 5.7 Markov point processes — 74
  - 5.7.1 Pairwise interaction point processes — 75
  - 5.7.2 More general forms of interaction — 78
- 5.8 Other constructions — 78
  - 5.8.1 Lattice-based processes — 78
  - 5.8.2 Thinned processes — 79
  - 5.8.3 Superpositions — 80
  - 5.8.4 Interactions in an inhomogeneous environment — 81
- 5.9 Multivariate models — 82

	5.9.1	Marked point processes	82
	5.9.2	Multivariate point processes	82
	5.9.3	How should multivariate models be formulated?	82
	5.9.4	Cox processes	83
	5.9.5	Markov point processes	85

6. Model-fitting using summary descriptions — 86
 6.1 Parameter estimation using the K-function — 86
  6.1.1 Least squares estimation — 86
  6.1.2 Illustration for simulations of a Poisson cluster process — 87
  6.1.3 Procedure when $K(t)$ is unknown — 88
 6.2 Goodness-of-fit assessment using nearest neighbour distributions — 89
 6.3 Examples — 90
  6.3.1 Redwood seedlings — 90
  6.3.2 Bramble canes — 92
 6.4 Parameter estimation via goodness-of-fit testing — 100
  6.4.1 Analysis of hamster tumour data — 100

7. Model-fitting using likelihood-based methods — 104
 7.1 Likelihood inference for inhomogeneous Poisson processes — 104
  7.1.1 Fitting a trend surface to the Lansing Woods data — 105
 7.2 Likelihood inference for Markov point processes — 107
  7.2.1 Maximum pseudo-likelihood estimation — 107
  7.2.2 Non-parametric estimation of a pairwise interaction function — 109
  7.2.3 Fitting a pairwise interaction point process to the displaced amacrine cells — 109
  7.2.4 Monte Carlo maximum likelihood estimation — 110
  7.2.5 The displaced amacrine cells revisited — 113
 7.3 Further reading — 114

8. Non-parametric methods — 115
 8.1 Estimating weighted integrals of the second-order intensity — 115
 8.2 Non-parametric estimation of a spatially varying intensities — 116
  8.2.1 Estimating spatially varying intensity for the Lansing Woods data — 118
 8.3 Analysing replicated spatial point patterns — 121
  8.3.1 Estimating the K-function from replicated data — 123
  8.3.2 Between-group comparisons in designed experiments — 124
  8.3.3 Parametric or non-parametric methods? — 127

9. Point process methods in spatial epidemiology — 128
 9.1 Introduction — 128
 9.2 Spatial clustering — 130
  9.2.1 Analysis of the North Humberside childhood leukaemia data — 131
  9.2.2 Other tests of spatial clustering — 132
 9.3 Spatial variation in risk — 133
 9.4 Point source models — 134
  9.4.1 Childhood asthma in North Derbyshire, England — 137
  9.4.2 Cancers in North Liverpool — 137

9.5		Stratification and matching	139
	9.5.1	Stratified case–control designs	139
	9.5.2	Individually matched case–control designs	141
	9.5.3	Is stratification or matching helpful?	143
9.6		Disentangling heterogeneity and clustering	143

References   **145**

Index   **155**

Preface

A spatial point pattern is a set of locations, irregularly distributed within a designated region and presumed to have been generated by some form of stochastic mechanism. In most applications, the designated region is essentially planar (two-dimensional Euclidean space), but one-dimensional applications are also possible, and three-dimensional applications are becoming more common in conjunction with the development of more sophisticated three-dimensional scanning microscopes. The first edition of *Statistical Analysis of Spatial Point Patterns* appeared in 1983. Its aim was to cover the major methodological themes of the subject and their application to data arising in the biological sciences, especially ecology.

In this second edition I have extended the methodological discussion to cover major developments in the intervening years, but have also tried to preserve the applied flavour of the book. Much of the newer work in the area tends to be mathematically sophisticated. My aim in covering this material has been to discuss the central ideas without going into the full technical detail which a rigorous treatment would require, and which is given in the original articles. I have also resisted the temptation to discuss spatial statistics more widely. Cressie (1991) identifies three major branches of spatial statistics, namely geostatistics, lattice processes and spatial point processes. Whilst these three topics are to some extent interlinked, they nevertheless give rise to distinct stochastic models and associated statistical methods, and can therefore be studied separately.

Within the realm of spatial point processes, perhaps the most important recent theoretical development has been the provision of formal, likelihood-based methods of inference for a reasonably wide range of models. These have partially replaced the more *ad hoc* methods which prevailed in the early 1980s. Nevertheless, some of the *ad hoc* methods remain useful, and have themselves been extended in various ways, for example in the adaptation of non-parametric smoothing methods to spatial point processes. New applications have also emerged and, as is usual in statistics, have in turn motivated further methodological development. The two new areas of application on which I draw most heavily are microanatomy and epidemiology.

In microanatomy, the points in an observed pattern typically are reference locations for cells in a microscopic tissue section. The underlying cellular structure influences the kinds of models which are appropriate, usually involving the concept of interactions between near-neighbouring cells. Perhaps more fundamentally from a statistical viewpoint, most microanatomical studies use a replicated sampling design in which data are obtained from several subjects and/or several tissue sections per subject, in contrast to the traditional emphasis throughout spatial statistics on the analysis of unreplicated patterns.

In epidemiology, the points are reference locations (typically place of residence) for cases of a disease in a geographical region, often supplemented by the reference locations for a set of controls sampled from the underlying population at risk. The principal methodological challenge in this area of application is to use the case–control paradigm to circumvent the obvious difficulty of building credible parametric models for human population distributions in a heterogeneous environment.

When the first edition was written, there were few other books available on the then emerging subject of spatial statistics, and none at all which dealt exclusively with the statistical analysis of spatial point patterns. A number of texts in spatial statistics are now available which contain substantial material on spatial point patterns. These include Ripley (1981), the two volumes of Upton and Fingleton (1985, 1989), Cliff and Ord (1981), Cressie (1991), Bailey and Gatrell (1995) and Stoyan *et al.* (1995). Matérn (1986) is a reissue of Bertil Matérn's classic 1960 Swedish doctoral dissertation. Van Lieshout (2000) deals exclusively with Markov point processes and their statistical analysis.

Inevitably, some topics which seemed important at the begining of the 1980s seem less so twenty years later, and the balance of the treatment of different topics in this second edition has changed accordingly. I have also corrected a number of errors in the first edition.

Public-domain data-sets and software can be downloaded from the author's web page:

http://www.maths.lancs.ac.uk/~diggle

Additional comments about software can be found at the end of Chapter 1.

My thanks are due to my colleagues, in Lancaster and elsewhere, who have provided me with such a stimulating working environment. Many have collaborated with me on jointly authored publications and should share the credit for whatever value the book may have, whereas responsibility for defects remains mine alone.

PETER J. DIGGLE
Lancaster
November 17, 2002

1
Introduction

1.1 Spatial point patterns

Data in the form of a set of points, irregularly distributed within a region of space, arise in many different contexts; examples include locations of trees in a forest, of nests in a breeding colony of birds, or of nuclei in a microscopic section of tissue. We call any such data-set a *spatial point pattern* and refer to the locations as *events*, to distinguish these from arbitrary points of the region in question.

Figures 1.1 and 1.2 show two spatial point patterns in a square region. The first, due to Numata (1961), shows 65 Japanese black pine saplings in a square of side 5.7 metres whilst the second, extracted by Ripley (1977) from Strauss (1975), shows 62 redwood seedlings in a square of side approximately 23 m. The two patterns appear strikingly different. Figure 1.1 shows no obvious structure and might be regarded as a 'completely random' pattern, in a sense which we shall define formally in due course. In Figure 1.2, on the other hand, the strong clustering of seedlings requires some biological explanation which, in this instance, is readily available. The seedlings cluster around redwood stumps which are known to be present in the study region, but whose locations have not been recorded. It is important to recognize that patterns like Figure 1.2 can arise either through some form of clustering mechanism or through

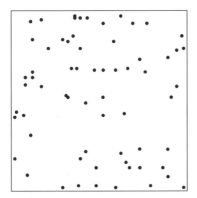

Figure 1.1. Locations of 65 Japanese black pine saplings in a square of side 5.7 metres (Numata, 1961).

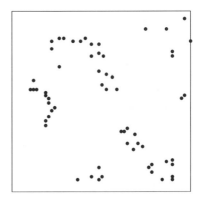

Figure 1.2. Locations of 62 redwood seedlings in a square of side 23 metres (Strauss, 1975; Ripley, 1977).

2 Statistical analysis of spatial point patterns

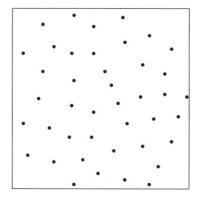

Figure 1.3. Locations of 42 cell centres in a unit square (Ripley, 1977).

environmental variation leading to local patches with relatively high concentrations of events. Here, as elsewhere, failure to record relevant biological information limits the conclusions which can be drawn from a statistical analysis. We therefore describe patterns like Figure 1.2 as 'aggregated' to avoid the mechanistic connotations of the perhaps more obvious term 'clustered'.

Figure 1.3 shows a further qualitatively different type of pattern, formed in this case by the centres of 42 biological cells (Crick and Lawrence, 1975; Ripley, 1977). The cell centres are distributed more or less regularly over the unit square, improbably so unless there is some associated regulating mechanism operating to encourage an even spatial distribution of cell centres. A possible explanation is that the cell centres are merely convenient reference points for cells whose physical size is non-negligible relative to the scale of observation. Quite generally, and again without wishing to imply any specific causal mechanism, we refer to such patterns as 'regular'.

The nature of the pattern generated by a biological process can be affected by the physical scale on which the process is observed. At a sufficiently large scale most natural environments exhibit heterogeneity, which will tend to produce aggregated patterns. At a smaller scale, environmental variation will be less pronounced and the major determinant of pattern may then be the nature of the interactions amongst the events themselves. For example, vegetative propagation of individual shoots will tend to produce small-scale aggregation whereas competition for space will encourage regularity. Our classification of patterns as regular, random or aggregated is therefore an oversimplification, but a useful one at an early stage of analysis. At a later stage, this simplistic approach can be abandoned in favour of a more detailed, and essentially multidimensional, description of pattern which can be obtained either by the use of a variety of functional summary statistics or by formulating an explicit model of the underlying process. The approach taken in this book will be to develop methods for the analysis of spatial patterns based on *stochastic models*, which assume that the events are generated by some underlying random mechanism.

Our fourth example, shown in Figure 1.4, introduces the idea of a *multivariate* point pattern. In this example, the points represent cells of two different types (hence, *bivariate*) in the retina of a rabbit. The data consist of the locations of 294 displaced amacrine cells, amongst which 152 are of a type which transmit information to the

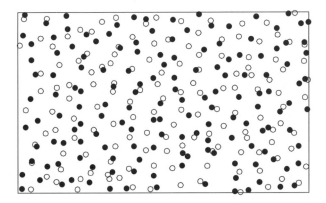

Figure 1.4. Locations of 294 displaced amacrine cells in the retina of a rabbit. Solid and open circles respectively identify on and off cells.

brain when a light goes *on*, whilst the remaining 142 transmit information when a light goes *off*. The relationship between the two component patterns can help to explain the developmental processes which operate within the immature retina. We shall re-examine the data from this point of view in Section 4.7.

We shall assume throughout this book that the region in question is essentially planar, although most of the ideas extend, at least in principle, to other dimensions. Even in one dimension, the distinction between temporal and spatial point patterns is important. In the case of series of events irregularly distributed in time, for example division times in a cell proliferation process, stochastic models and their associated statistical methods reflect the essentially unidirectional quality of the time dimension, whereas in the corresponding spatial case, for example nesting sites along the bank of a canal, no such directionality exists. Cox and Lewis (1966) give an excellent introduction to the analysis of temporal point patterns.

We confine our attention to applications in the biological sciences, broadly interpreted to include biomedicine and epidemiology, although similar problems arise in many other disciplines. For examples in archaeology, astronomy and geography see, respectively, Hodder and Orton (1976), Peebles (1974) and Cliff and Ord (1981). To some extent, the methods which we describe remain useful (and have certainly been used) in these other areas of application, but should not be adopted uncritically. In particular, our stochastic models will be motivated by simple considerations of possible underlying biological mechanisms which may or may not be relevant in other disciplines.

1.2 Sampling

The selection of the study region, A say, merits some discussion. In some applications, A is objectively determined by the problem in hand, and inferences are required in terms of a process defined on A itself. One example of this would be a map of all nesting sites on an island. More commonly, A is selected from some much larger region. The selection of A may then be made according to a probability sampling scheme, or it may simply reflect the experimenter's view that A is in some sense representative of the larger region. In either case, but particularly the latter, inferences drawn from an analysis will carry much greater conviction if consistency over replicate data-sets can be demonstrated.

As an alternative to intensive mapping within a single region A, the experimenter may choose to record limited information from a large number of smaller regions, for example the number of events in each region. In this context, the regions are called *quadrats* and the data are referred to as *quadrat counts*. A quadrat was originally a square of side 1 metre, used by the Uppsala school of plant ecologists as the basic sampling unit for investigating plant communities in the field (Du Rietz, 1929).

Quadrat sampling remains a popular field technique in plant ecology and elsewhere, but in some contexts it is rather impractical and this has led to the development, initially in the American forestry literature (Cottam and Curtis, 1949), of a number of *distance methods* for sampling spatial point patterns. In these, the basic sampling unit is a point, and information is recorded in the form of distances to neighbouring events, for example the distances to the first few nearest events.

We shall refer to quadrat count and distance methods as *sparse sampling* methods, to distinguish them from intensive mapping exercises. It turns out that the appropriate techniques for the analysis of data obtained by sparse sampling and by intensive mapping are quite different. Also, analyses of sparsely sampled patterns typically have more limited objectives than do analyses of mapped patterns.

A particular form of quadrat sampling, intermediate between sparse sampling and intensive mapping, consists of partitioning the study region into disjoint sub-regions and recording the number of events in each sub-region. Data of this kind arise in two very different ways. The first, which has a long tradition as a method of field sampling in plant ecology, is when a rectangular study region is partitioned into a regular grid of square or rectangular quadrats, and a count is taken within each quadrat. See, for example, Greig and Smith (1964) or Kershaw (1973). The second, which typically arises in environmental epidemiology, is when health outcome data are routinely maintained as counts of the numbers of events in administratively defined sub-regions. In either case, the resulting data can be represented as a realization of a high-dimensional multivariate random variable, $Y = (Y_1, \ldots, Y_n)$ say, where Y_i denotes the number of events in the ith sub-region. In this setting, a stochastic model for the underlying point process would induce a unique statistical distribution on Y, but in practice the form of this distribution tends to be intractable except in a few special cases. A pragmatic alternative is to formulate a model directly for the distribution of Y, without reference to any underlying point process. The usual method of construction is to specify the set of conditional distributions of each Y_i given all other Y_j. Models of this kind are called *Markov random fields*. Their construction must satisfy sometimes non-obvious constraints to ensure self-consistency. For an early, and very influential, account, see Besag (1974).

Replicated sampling of mapped patterns has been surprisingly rare until quite recently. Ecological investigations have certainly compared patterns in study regions deliberately selected to represent different environmental conditions, but I am not aware of corresponding studies which have been designed with a view to establishing the consistency of patterns in ostensibly similar regions. Pseudo-replication can always be achieved by partitioning a single region into two or more sub-regions, and is sometimes useful. Genuine replication has become more common with the adoption of spatial point pattern methods for the analysis of microanatomical images (see, for example, Baddeley *et al.*, 1993). In this context, each study region A represents a single field of view under a microscope, and there is a well-established tradition of using hierarchical sampling designs of the form: multiple fields of view within tissue sections; multiple tissue sections within subjects; multiple subjects within experimental treatment groups. Studies of this kind lend themselves to design-based inference as an alternative to the more widely prevailing model-based inference for spatial point patterns.

1.3 Edge effects

Edge effects arise in spatial point pattern analysis when, as is often the case in practice, the region A on which the pattern is observed is part of a larger region on which the underlying process operates. The essential difficulty is that unobserved events outside A may interact with observed events within A but, precisely because the events in question are not observed, it is difficult to take proper account of this.

For some kinds of exploratory analysis, edge effects can safely be ignored. We shall discuss when and why this is so at appropriate points in the text. More generally, we can distinguish between three broad approaches to handling edge effects: the use of buffer zones; explicit adjustments to take account of unobserved events; and, when A is rectangular, wrapping A onto a torus by identifying opposite edges. We will illustrate each of these approaches by considering a statistic which arises in several contexts, namely the number of events which occur within a specified distance of an arbitrary event or location.

The buffer zone method consists of carrying out all aspects of the statistical analysis after conditioning on the locations of all events which fall within a buffer zone B consisting of all points less than a specified distance, d_0 say, from the edge of A. Let $C = A - B$ denote the remainder of A after subtracting the buffer zone. Then it is clear that for any event or location $x \in C$, the *observed* number of events within a distance d of x must equal the actual number of events *in the underlying process* within distance d of x, provided $d \leq d_0$, whereas for $d > d_0$ the observed number may be less than the actual number, thereby biasing any estimates based on these observed numbers. The choice of d_0 in the buffer zone method is awkward, since too small a value leaves residual edge effects, whereas too large a value effectively throws away data unnecessarily. However, the method can be applied in adaptive form, varying the value of d_0 according to the particular statistic being used.

The adjustment method operates by making an 'on average' adjustment for the unobserved events outside A. Again using our simple example to illustrate, if we count the observed number, n say, of events within distance d of a location x, and $a(d)$ denotes the area of intersection between A and a disc of radius d centred on the location x, then an intuitively sensible estimate of the actual number of events within distance d of x is $n\pi d^2/a(d)$. The adjustment method is attractive because it makes full use of the observed data, especially when relatively large-scale effects are of interest. Note, however, that the adjustments typically lead to an increased sampling variance for the edge-adjusted estimator by comparison with its unadjusted counterpart. In essence, this is an example of the common trade-off in statistical estimation between bias and variance; edge corrections seek to eliminate bias at the expense of some increase in variance.

Toroidal wrapping of a rectangular A is not so much an edge-correction method as a trick to eliminate edge effects in particular circumstances. Its most common use is as a convenient way of simulating realizations of various kinds of point process. For example, suppose that we wish to simulate a point process model for the cell centre data shown in Figure 1.3, the most obvious feature of which is that no two events can occur too close together. If we attempt to simulate a process of this kind directly on a unit square A, then points near the edge of A are favoured over points near the centre of A as potential locations, because of the absence of potentially inhibiting events outside A. By simulating the process on a torus and subsequently unwrapping to a unit square for presentation, we avoid this effect. Note that it will seldom make sense to wrap observed data onto a torus for analysis; for example, if we were to do this with the cell centre data, then we would observe some very small toroidal distances between pairs of cells, thus destroying the essential inhibitory nature of the underlying process.

1.4 Complete spatial randomness

The hypothesis of *complete spatial randomness* (CSR) for a spatial point pattern asserts that (i) the number of events in any planar region A with area $|A|$ follows a Poisson distribution with mean $\lambda|A|$; (ii) given n events x_i in a region A, the x_i are an independent random sample from the uniform distribution on A. The self-consistency of (i) and (ii) is not immediately obvious, but will be established in Chapter 4. In (i), the constant λ is the *intensity*, or mean number of events per unit area. According to (i), CSR therefore implies that the intensity of events does not vary over the plane. According to (ii), CSR also implies that there are no interactions amongst the events. For example, the independence assumption in (ii) would be violated if the existence of an event at x either encouraged or inhibited the occurrence of other events in the neighbourhood of x. In developing tests of CSR for sparsely sampled patterns the starting point will be property (i), whilst for mapped patterns it is more usual to start with (ii), i.e. to analyse the pattern conditional on the observed number of events.

Intuitive ideas about what constitutes a 'random pattern' can be misleading. Figure 1.5 shows a realization of 100 events independently and uniformly distributed

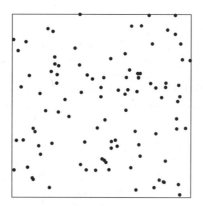

Figure 1.5. Realization of CSR: 100 events in a unit square.

on the unit square. Any visual impression of aggregation is illusory. Note also the superficial similarity to Figure 1.1.

Our interest in CSR is that it represents an idealized standard which, if strictly unattainable in practice, may nevertheless be tenable as a convenient first approximation. Most analyses begin with a test of CSR, and there are several good reasons for this. Firstly, a pattern for which CSR is not rejected scarcely merits any further formal statistical analysis. Secondly, tests are used as a means of exploring a set of data, rather than because rejection of CSR is of intrinsic interest. Greig-Smith, in the discussion of Bartlett (1971), has emphasized that ecologists often know CSR to be untenable but nevertheless use tests of CSR as aids to the formulation of ecologically interesting hypotheses concerning pattern and its genesis. Thirdly, CSR acts as a dividing hypothesis to distinguish between patterns which are broadly classifiable as 'regular' or 'aggregated'.

Another use of CSR is as a building block in the construction of more complex models. We shall return to this topic in Chapter 5.

1.5 Objectives of statistical analysis

In any particular application, the objectives of a statistical analysis should be determined by the scientist's objectives in collecting the data in question. We have already given reasons for beginning an analysis with a test of CSR. What to do next will vary according to context.

In sparse sampling exercises, a specific objective may be to estimate the intensity. For example, in forestry surveys an important quantity to be estimated is the 'stocking density', or number of stems per hectare. The nature of the pattern might then be of interest only inasmuch as it affects the sampling distribution of the estimator.

With mapped data, the scientist will usually want a more detailed description of the observed pattern than can be provided by a test of CSR. One way to achieve this is by formulating a parametric stochastic model and fitting it to the data. If a model can be found which fits the data well, the estimated values of its parameters provide summary statistics which can be used to compare ostensibly similar data-sets. More ambitiously, a fitted model can provide an explanation of the underlying scientific processes. But this must involve an element of *non-statistical* inference: quite apart from the obvious fact that a model which fits the data is not necessarily correct in any absolute sense, we shall see in Chapter 4 that a simple stochastic model for a spatial point pattern may admit of more than one scientific interpretation.

Of course, it is generally the case that modelling itself is only a means to a wider end. A well-formulated, and well-fitting, model provides a parsimonious description of a complex pattern, and one which will be especially useful if its parameters can be related to scientific hypotheses about the underlying phenomenon being studied.

Model-fitting is particularly difficult for large, heterogeneous data-sets. In such cases, it may be unhelpful to force a parametric analysis based on untenable assumptions. For example, a generic problem in environmental epidemiology is to estimate the spatial variation in the risk of a particular disease, using data on the locations of individual cases in a geographical region. One approach to this problem might be to formulate an idealized model for the observed spatial pattern of cases under the assumption that risk is spatially constant, and to investigate deviations of the observed pattern from this model. An alternative, which would be more in line with classical

8 Statistical analysis of spatial point patterns

epidemiological methods, would be to make a non-parametric comparison between the pattern of cases and a second pattern of *controls*, defined to be a random sample from the population at risk. We shall discuss this idea in detail in Chapter 9.

1.6 The Dirichlet tessellation

Given n distinct events x_i in a planar region A, we can assign to x_i a 'territory' consisting of that part of A which is closer to x_i than to any other x_j. This construction, referred to either as the *Dirichlet tessellation* or the *Voronoi tessellation* of the events in A, has been incorporated into stochastic models of natural phenomena such as inter-plant competition. In these models, plants whose territories abut are assumed to be in direct competition for available nutrient; see, for example, Cormack (1979, pp. 171–5). For large n, the tessellation is also the basis of a computationally efficient solution to a number of problems involving the calculation of distances between events.

Except possibly along the boundary of A, each territory or *cell* is a convex polygonal region. Events x_i and x_j whose cells share a common boundary segment are said to be *contiguous*. Typically, each cell vertex is common to three cells, and the lines joining the pairs of contiguous events define a triangulation of the x_i, called the *Delaunay triangulation*. Thus, cell boundaries can be obtained as the perpendicular bisectors of the edges of the triangulation, and cell vertices are the corresponding circumcentres. Figure 1.6 shows a simple example of both the tessellation and the triangulation associated with $n = 12$ events in a unit square. Rogers (1964) discusses the mathematical properties of the Dirichlet tessellation in a general p-dimensional setting.

The construction of the Dirichlet tessellation and the associated Delaunay triangulation rapidly becomes a non-trivial exercise as n increases. Green and Sibson (1978) give a remarkably efficient algorithm whose computational cost increases roughly as $n^{1.5}$.

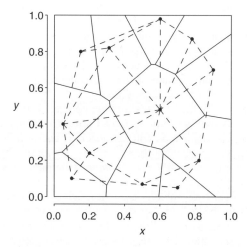

Figure 1.6. The Dirichlet tessellation (solid lines) and Delaunay triangulation (dashed lines) associated with 12 points in a unit square.

1.7 Monte Carlo tests

Even simple stochastic models for spatial point patterns lead to intractable distribution theory, and in order to test models against data we shall make extensive use of Monte Carlo tests (Barnard, 1963).

Quite generally, let u_1 be the observed value of a statistic U and let $u_i : i = 2, \ldots, s$, be corresponding values generated by independent random sampling from the distribution of U under a simple hypothesis $\mathcal{H}$. Let $u_{(j)}$ denote the jth largest amongst $u_i : i = 1, \ldots, s$. Then, under $\mathcal{H}$,

$$P\{u_1 = u_{(j)}\} = s^{-1} : j = 1, \ldots, s,$$

and rejection of $\mathcal{H}$ on the basis that u_1 ranks kth largest or higher gives an exact, one-sided test of size k/s. This assumes that the values of the u_i are all different, so that the ranking of u_1 is unambiguous. If U is a discrete random variable, for example a count, tied values are possible and we then adopt the conservative rule of choosing the least extreme rank for u_1. The extension to two-sided tests is clear.

Hope (1968) gives a number of examples to show that the loss of power resulting from a Monte Carlo implementation is slight, so that s need not be very large. For a one-sided test at the conventional 5% level, $s = 100$ is adequate.

Power loss is related to Marriott's (1979) investigation of 'blurred critical regions', which arise because a value of u_1 which would be declared significant in a classical test may not be declared significant in a Monte Carlo test, and vice versa. Let the (unknown) distribution function of U under $\mathcal{H}$ be $F(u)$. For a one-sided 5% test with $s = 20k$, the probability that we reject $\mathcal{H}$, given that $U = u_1$, is

$$p(u_1) = \sum_{r=0}^{k-1} \binom{s-1}{r} \{1 - F(u_1)\}^r \{F(u_1)\}^{s-1-r}. \tag{1.1}$$

For a classical test, represented here by the limit $s \to \infty$, $p(u_1)$ is 1 or 0 accordingly as $F(u_1)$ is greater or less than 0.95. The effect of the 'blurring' introduced by (1.1) is measured by Marriott's Table 1, here represented by Figure 1.7. Marriott concludes also that the extent of the blurring depends primarily on k, so that if $s = 100$ is judged to be acceptable for a test at the 5% level, then $s = 500$ should be used for a test at the 1% level, and pro rata for tests at smaller levels. These recommended values of s are smaller than would be considered adequate for the estimation of $P\{U > u_1 \mid \mathcal{H}\}$. This is essentially a consequence of the blurring effect: it is the *rank* of u_1, and not u_1 itself, which is the test statistic.

A technical point concerning the use of Monte Carlo tests is that in practice random sampling will be replaced by pseudo-random sampling. At different times, we have used the generator supplied in the NAG (1977) subroutine library, a Fortran implementation of the Wichmann and Hill (1982) generator and the S-Plus function `runif()` (Venables and Ripley, 1994). Other references for users who need to provide their own generator include Kennedy and Gentle (1980) and Ripley (1987).

A more subtle, but potentially more important, criticism is that Monte Carlo tests encourage 'data-dredging', since the user can choose the statistic U to focus on any seemingly aberrant feature of their data. Whilst we admit that this is a danger, it should be obvious that 'significant' results based on pathological test statistics are of no practical value.

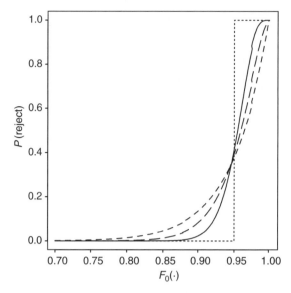

Figure 1.7. Blurred critical regions for one-sided 5% Monte Carlo tests with $s=20$ (shorter-dashed curve), 40 (longer-dashed curve), 100 (solid curve) and $s\to\infty$ (dotted curve) (adapted from Marriott, 1979).

An inherent weakness of the Monte Carlo approach is its restriction to simple hypotheses $\mathcal{H}$. Composite hypotheses can be tested if pseudo-random sampling is made conditional on the observed values of sufficient statistics for any unknown parameters, but this is seldom practicable. Note that a goodness-of-fit test which ignores the effects of estimating parameters will tend to be conservative. This particular difficulty does not arise with tests of CSR for mapped data, because the observed number of events n is sufficient for the intensity λ, and, conditional on n, CSR is a simple hypothesis. But it does affect the assessment of goodness of fit for more general stochastic models. An approximate remedy, which we discuss further in Chapter 6, is to measure goodness of fit by a statistic which is not directly related to the procedure used to estimate the parameters of the model.

The principal advantage to be set against the above is that the investigator need not be constrained by known distribution theory, but rather can and should use informative statistics of their own choosing.

When asymptotic distribution theory is available, Monte Carlo testing provides an exact alternative for small samples and a useful check on the applicability of the asymptotic theory. If the results of classical and Monte Carlo tests are in substantial agreement, little or nothing has been lost; if not, the explanation is usually that the classical test uses inappropriate distributional assumptions.

1.8 Software

Spatial point pattern analysis is computationally intensive, not least because of the heavy reliance on Monte Carlo methods of inference. The S-Plus spatial statistics module (Kaluzny *et al.*, 1996) offers some, but not all, of the required functionality. The Splancs library (Rowlingson and Diggle, 1993) gives a wider range of functions for statistical analysis and is more flexible in other ways; for example, it can handle data on arbitrary polygonal regions. The Spatstat library, written by Adrian Baddeley and Rolf Turner, also implements a wide range of methods, with a stronger emphasis than Splancs on parametric modelling.

The analyses reported in this book were implemented using a combination of Splancs, Spatstat and Voronoi (a package for computation of the Dirichlet tessellation, written by Rolf Turner), together with some additional functions written by the author.

More sophisticated displays than those shown in this book, for example colour-coded overlays of point pattern maps and contour maps, can most easily be produced using a geographical information system (GIS). There is an S-Plus interface to at least one widely used proprietary GIS, Arc-Info.

An extremely useful recent development has been the growth of the R software system. This is very similar in style to S-Plus, but with the crucial difference that it is freely available. Many add-on libraries of R functions are also available. In particular, R versions of Splancs, Spatstat and Voronoi are available. For further information about R, a good starting point is the R website, http://www.r-project.org

2
Preliminary testing

2.1 Tests of complete spatial randomness

Although complete spatial randomness is of limited scientific interest in itself, there are several good reasons why we might begin an analysis with a test of CSR: rejection of CSR is a minimal prerequisite to any serious attempt to model an observed pattern; tests are used to explore a set of data and to assist in the formulation of plausible alternatives to CSR; CSR operates as a dividing hypothesis between regular and aggregated patterns.

In view of the above, the present discussion emphasizes two aspects: the value of graphical methods, which will almost always be informative and will sometimes make formal testing unnecessary; and informal combination of several complementary tests, to indicate the nature of any departure from CSR. With regard to the second of these, if a single assessment of significance is required the following result is useful. Suppose that the attained significance levels of k not necessarily independent tests of CSR are $p_j : j = 1, \ldots, k$ and let $p_{\min}$ be the smallest such p_j, corresponding to the most significant departure from CSR. Then, under CSR,

$$p \leq P\{p_{\min} \leq p\} \leq kp. \tag{2.1}$$

For k independent tests, the exact result is

$$P\{p_{\min} \leq p\} = 1 - (1-p)^k.$$

Cox (1977) points out that using multiple tests as part of a diagnostic procedure makes practical sense only if the various tests examine different aspects of pattern, so that a significant result for one test does not prevent a sensible interpretation of the others.

We acknowledge that testing complete spatial randomness is a very unambitious agenda in itself, and should be seen as no more than a natural starting point. From a pedagogical point of view, it provides a historical perspective on the early development of the subject, and an opportunity to illustrate a number of general issues in the simplest possible setting. These include the role of Monte Carlo methods, the need to assess the relative merits of intuitively sensible but *ad hoc* methods and, perhaps most importantly, the need to take account of the inherent dependence amongst multiple measurements derived from a single point pattern. In the remainder of the chapter we will therefore describe a number of different tests which have been proposed, and assess their strengths and weaknesses. As illustrative examples, we shall use repeatedly the three data-sets shown in Figures 1.1–1.3, each of which has a straightforward

2.2 Inter-event distances

One possible summary description of a pattern of n events in a region A is the empirical distribution of the $\frac{1}{2}n(n-1)$ inter-event distances, t_{ij} say. The corresponding theoretical distribution of the distance T between two events independently and uniformly distributed in A depends on the size and shape of A, but is expressible in closed form for the most common cases of square or circular A (Bartlett, 1964).

For A a square of unit side, the distribution function of T is

$$H(t) = \begin{cases} \pi t^2 - 8t^3/3 + t^4/2 & : 0 \le t \le 1 \\ 1/3 - 2t^2 - t^4/2 + 4(t^2-1)^{\frac{1}{2}}(2t^2+1)/3 \\ \quad + 2t^2 \sin^{-1}(2t^{-2}-1) & : 1 < t \le \sqrt{2} \end{cases} \quad (2.2)$$

whilst for a circle of unit radius the corresponding expression is

$$H(t) = 1 + \pi^{-1}\{2(t^2-1)\cos^{-1}(t/2) - t(1+t^2/2)\sqrt{(1-t^2/4)}\} \quad (2.3)$$

for all $0 \le t \le 2$.

We now develop a test of CSR based specifically on inter-event distances; the general approach is applicable to other summary descriptions and will reappear in later sections.

Assume that for the particular region A in question, $H(t)$ is known. Calculate the empirical distribution function (EDF) of inter-event distances. This function, $\hat{H}_1(t)$ say, represents the observed proportion of inter-event distances t_{ij} which are at most t; thus,

$$\hat{H}_1(t) = \{\tfrac{1}{2}n(n-1)\}^{-1} \#(t_{ij} \le t),$$

where # means 'the number of'. Now prepare a plot of $\hat{H}_1(t)$ as ordinate against $H(t)$ as abscissa. If the data are compatible with CSR, the plot should be roughly linear. To assess the significance or otherwise of departures from linearity, the conventional approach would be to find the sampling distribution of $\hat{H}_1(t)$ under CSR, but this is complicated by the dependence between inter-event distances with a common end-point, and we therefore proceed as follows. Calculate EDFs $\hat{H}_i(t) : i = 2, 3, \ldots, s$, from each of $s-1$ independent simulations of n events independently and uniformly distributed on A, and define *upper* and *lower simulation envelopes*,

$$U(t) = \max\{\hat{H}_i(t)\}, \quad (2.4)$$

$$L(t) = \min\{\hat{H}_i(t)\}. \quad (2.5)$$

where in each case, i runs from 2 to s. These simulation envelopes can also be plotted against $H(t)$, and have the property that under CSR, and for each t,

$$P\{\hat{H}_1(t) > U(t)\} = P\{\hat{H}_1(t) < L(t)\} = s^{-1}. \quad (2.6)$$

14 *Statistical analysis of spatial point patterns*

The simulation envelopes are intended to help in the interpretation of the plot of $\hat{H}_1(t)$ against $H(t)$, and we shall shortly give examples of their use. Two of the many possible approaches to the construction of an exact Monte Carlo test of CSR are as follows.

(i) Choose t_0 and define $u_i = \hat{H}_i(t_0)$. As described in Section 1.7, the rank of u_1 amongst the u_i provides the basis of a test because under CSR all rankings of u_1 are equiprobable.
(ii) Define u_i to be a measure of the discrepancy between $\hat{H}_i(t)$ and $H(t)$ over the whole range of t, for example

$$u_i = \int \{\hat{H}_i(t) - H(t)\}^2 \, dt \qquad (2.7)$$

and again proceed to a test based on the rank of u_1.

The first approach makes sense only if t_0 can be chosen in a way which is natural to the problem in hand. The second has the advantage of objectivity but we shall see that in the particular context of inter-event distances it often gives a very weak test. In any event, no single test statistic should be allowed to override a critical inspection of the EDF plot.

If the region A is one for which the theoretical distribution function $H(t)$ is unknown, a test can still be carried out if, in (2.7), $H(t)$ is replaced by

$$\bar{H}_i(t) = (s-1)^{-1} \sum_{j \neq i} \hat{H}_j(t).$$

The u_i are no longer independent under CSR, but are exchangeable and the required property that under CSR all rankings of u_1 are equiprobable therefore still holds. Similarly, the graphical procedure then consists of plotting $\hat{H}_1(t)$, $U(t)$ and $L(t)$ against $\bar{H}_1(t)$. Note that because $\bar{H}_1(t)$ involves only the simulations of CSR and not the original data, it provides an unbiased estimate of $H(t)$ under the null hypothesis.

2.2.1 Analysis of Japanese black pine saplings

Figure 2.1 shows the plot of $\hat{H}_1(t)$, $U(t)$ and $L(t)$ against $H(t)$ for Numata's data previously given as Figure 1.1. Note that $\hat{H}_1(t)$ lies close to $H(t)$ and between $U(t)$ and $L(t)$ throughout its range, which suggests acceptance of CSR. A formal test based on the integrated squared difference (2.7) and 99 simulations ($s = 100$) leads to an attained significance level of 0.37, and we conclude that these data are compatible with a completely random spatial distribution of saplings over the study region. The same conclusion was reached by Bartlett (1964) and by Besag and Diggle (1977), who based their test on Pearson's X^2 goodness-of-fit statistic applied to a histogram of inter-event distances.

2.2.2 Analysis of redwood seedlings

For the redwood data of Figure 1.2, a test based on (2.7) again suggests acceptance of CSR with an attained significance level of 0.22, but a detailed inspection of the EDF

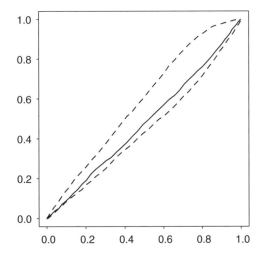

Figure 2.1. EDF plot of inter-event distances for Japanese black pine saplings: data (solid curve); upper and lower envelopes from 99 simulations of CSR (dashed curves).

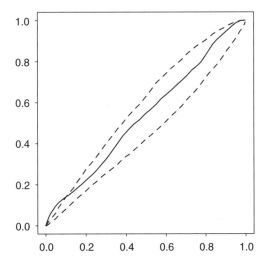

Figure 2.2. EDF plot of inter-event distances for redwood seedlings: data (solid curve); upper and lower envelopes from 99 simulations of CSR (dashed curves).

plot in Figure 2.2 leads to a different conclusion. We see that $\hat{H}_1(t)$ is greater than $H(t)$ throughout its range and in particular is greater than $U(t)$ for both very small and very large values of $H(t)$. The excess of small inter-event distances is compatible with an underlying clustering mechanism for which, as we have seen, there is a ready biological explanation. Further reinforcement of this conclusion, if any were needed, lies in Strauss's remark that a distance of 6 feet (approximately 2 metres) on the ground, corresponding to $t \approx 0.08$, 'was thought to be very roughly the range at which a pair

16 *Statistical analysis of spatial point patterns*

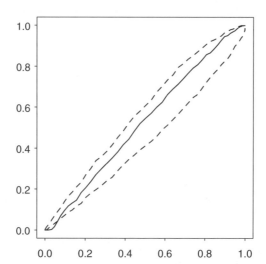

Figure 2.3. EDF plot of inter-event distances for biological cells: data (solid curve); upper and lower envelopes from 99 simulations of CSR (dashed curves).

of seedlings could interact'. This suggests that $\hat{H}_1(0.08)$, the observed proportion of inter-event distances less than or equal to 6 feet, is a reasonable test statistic. Since $\hat{H}_1(0.08) > U(0.08)$, it follows that CSR is rejected at a (one-sided) attained significance level of 0.01. Strictly, of course, this conclusion would only be valid if we had chosen our test statistic to be $\hat{H}_1(0.08)$ before inspecting Figure 2.2. Perhaps a more useful message from this example is that it reinforces the value of looking at the EDF plot in conjunction with its simulation envelopes, rather than relying on the result of a formal test of significance.

2.2.3 Analysis of biological cells

For Ripley's cell data previously given as Figure 1.3, a test based on (2.7) again suggests acceptance of CSR, this time with an attained significance level of 0.23, but inspection of the EDF plot in Figure 2.3 again suggests otherwise. The most striking feature of this plot is the complete absence of small inter-event distances, so that $\hat{H}_1(t) = 0$ for small t. This provides an explanation for the regular appearance of the observed pattern. Also, at large values of $H(t)$ we see that $\hat{H}_1(t)$ lies close to, albeit below, $U(t)$. This is unusual for a regular pattern, and encourages us to re-examine Figure 1.3. With the benefit of hindsight we see a surprising lack of events in the corners of the unit square, which suggests that there may have been some difficulty in determining the boundary of the study region.

2.2.4 Small distances

For the redwood seedlings and the biological cells, the evidence against CSR derives from the excess or deficiency, respectively, of *small* inter-event distances. The main body of the distribution of inter-event distance is relatively insensitive to changes in pattern.

It follows that at larger values of t, departures from the null form of $H(t)$ are usually swamped by sampling fluctuations in $\hat{H}_1(t)$, unless n is very large. Thus, while the EDF plot is informative, the test based on (2.7) is not recommended.

An extreme case of concentrating on small inter-event distances would be to use as test statistic the minimum inter-event distance. This is theoretically attractive if regular alternatives to CSR are suspected, because for particular kinds of regular alternative to CSR it can be derived as a likelihood ratio statistic. Furthermore, an approximate test can be implemented without simulations. Silverman and Brown (1978) express the asymptotic null distribution of T_k, the kth smallest inter-event distance, as

$$n(n-1)\pi|A|^{-1}T_k^2 \sim \chi_{2k}^2. \tag{2.8}$$

Ripley and Silverman (1978) suggest that the chi-squared approximation is adequate for $k \leq 9$ when $n \geq 30$.

For the biological cells, the observed value of T_1, the minimum inter-event distance, is 0.086. With $n=42$ and $|A|=1$, (2.8) gives $P\{T_1 \geq 0.086\} < 0.000005$ and CSR is overwhelmingly rejected. The same test accepts CSR for both the Japanese black pines and the redwoods.

A disadvantage of this test for large data-sets is its sensitivity to recording inaccuracies. For example, suppose that n events in the unit square are mapped to an accuracy of two decimal places in each coordinate direction, which corresponds approximately to the accuracy achieved in Figures 1.1–1.3. Then, the observed value of T_1 must be either zero, and significantly small according to (2.8), or at least 0.01. From (2.8), we can deduce that the upper critical value of T_1 for a one-sided 5% test of CSR is approximately $1.38\{n(n-1)\}^{\frac{1}{2}}$, and this is *less* than 0.01 if $n \geq 139$. A test based on T_k for some value of $k > 1$ is more robust in this respect, but the choice of k then becomes rather arbitrary.

2.3 Nearest neighbour distances

For n events in a region A, let y_i denote the distance from the ith event to the nearest other event in A. The y_i are called nearest neighbour distances, and typically include duplicate measurements between reciprocal nearest neighbour pairs. We can calculate the EDF, $\hat{G}_1(y)$ say, of the nearest neighbour distances by analogy with the calculation used in Section 2.2 to obtain $\hat{H}_1(t)$. Thus,

$$\hat{G}_1(y) = n^{-1}\#(y_i \leq y).$$

In many practical situations, interactions between events exist, if at all, only at a small physical scale. For example, trees would be expected to compete for sunlight or nutrient within an area roughly confined to their crowns or root systems, respectively. In such cases, nearest neighbour distances provide an objective means of concentrating on 'small' inter-event distances when a precise threshold distance cannot be specified in advance.

The theoretical distribution of the nearest neighbour distance Y under CSR depends on n and on A, and is not expressible in closed form because of complicated edge effects. An approximation which ignores these edge effects is obtained by noting that if $|A|$ denotes the area of A, then $\pi y^2 |A|^{-1}$ is the probability under CSR that an arbitrary event is within distance y of a specified event. Since the events are located independently, the approximate distribution function of Y is

$$G(y) = 1 - (1 - \pi y^2 |A|^{-1})^{n-1}.$$

A further approximation for large n, writing $\lambda = n|A|^{-1}$, is

$$G(y) = 1 - \exp(-\lambda \pi y^2) : y \geq 0. \tag{2.9}$$

This result is well known, and we shall reach it by a different route in Chapter 3.

The EDF $\hat{G}_1(y)$ can be compared with upper and lower simulation envelopes from simulated EDFs $\hat{G}_i(y) : i = 2, \ldots, s$ exactly as in Section 2.2. The approximate result (2.9) can be used to suggest a suitable range of tabulation but, because it is approximate, it is generally preferable to use the sample mean $\bar{G}_1(y)$ of simulated EDFs for linearization of the EDF plot. Possible bases for a Monte Carlo test include the sample mean of the n nearest neighbour distances, or

$$u_i = \int \{\hat{G}_i(y) - \bar{G}_i(y)\}^2 \, dy. \tag{2.10}$$

In (2.10),

$$\bar{G}_i(y) = (s-1)^{-1} \sum_{j \neq i} \hat{G}_j(y)$$

is defined by analogy with $\bar{H}_i(t)$ in Section 2.2. A test based on the sample mean, $\bar{y}$, was proposed by Clark and Evans (1954), but without proper allowance for the dependencies amongst the nearest neighbour distances. One possible advantage of a test based on $\bar{y}$ is that, as with the test based on the minimum inter-event distance, simulation is unnecessary. Donnelly (1978) has shown that, to a good approximation, the distribution of $\bar{y}$ under CSR is Normal, with mean and variance

$$E[\bar{y}] = 0.5(n^{-1}|A|)^{1/2} + (0.051 + 0.042 n^{-1/2}) n^{-1} P \tag{2.11}$$

and

$$\mathrm{Var}(\bar{y}) = 0.070 n^{-2} |A| + 0.037 (n^{-5} |A|)^{1/2} P, \tag{2.12}$$

where P denotes the perimeter length of A. Significantly small or large values of $\bar{y}$ indicate aggregation or regularity, respectively. A minor qualification is that the approximations break down for very convoluted regions A, in which case a Monte Carlo implementation is again necessary. Also, we maintain that informal inspection of the EDF plot is at least as important as formal testing.

The obvious method of computing nearest neighbour distances involves a crude search through all the inter-event distances. For sufficiently large n a more efficient method is to construct the Dirichlet tessellation of the n events, and then to search for nearest neighbour distances within the tessellation. This exploits the fact that, however large n is, each event is contiguous to, on average, six other events, one of which must be its nearest neighbour. As a result, only a small fraction of the inter-event distances need to be calculated. Peter Green (personal communication) has shown that the crude

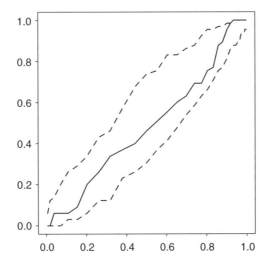

Figure 2.4. EDF plot of nearest neighbour distances for Japanese black pine saplings: data (solid curve); upper and lower envelopes from 99 simulations of CSR (dashed curves).

search is more efficient than the tessellation method for n less than about 500, but thereafter becomes progressively less efficient with increasing n.

2.3.1 Analysis of Japanese black pine saplings

Figure 2.4 shows the EDF plot of nearest neighbour distances for the Japanese black pine saplings, together with the upper and lower envelopes from 99 simulations of CSR. The plot suggests acceptance of CSR, as does a Monte Carlo test based on (2.10) with an attained significance level of 0.52. In addition the observed value of $\bar{y}$ is 0.0660, whilst (2.11) and (2.12) give $E[\bar{y}] = 0.0655$ and $\mathrm{Var}(\bar{y}) = 0.000021$, and hence a standard Normal deviate of -0.11, again suggesting acceptance of CSR.

Incidentally, and in contrast to Figures 2.1–2.3, the linear interpolation between values of the EDF calculated at intervals of 0.01 shows up clearly in Figure 2.4. However, the limited resolution of the data does not justify either a much finer tabulation or a more subtle interpolation rule.

2.3.2 Analysis of redwood seedlings

For the redwood seedlings, a Monte Carlo test based on (2.10) leads to emphatic rejection of CSR, with u_1 comfortably larger than all 99 simulated u_j. The EDF plot, Figure 2.5, clearly shows the excess of small nearest neighbour distances which is a characteristic feature of aggregated patterns. The observed value of $\bar{y}$ is 0.0385. This corresponds to a standard Normal deviate of -5.96 and again provides strong evidence for rejection of CSR in favour of an aggregated alternative.

2.3.3 Analysis of biological cells

For the biological cells, (2.10) again gives a value of u_1 which is comfortably larger than all 99 simulated values u_j, whilst the EDF plot, Figure 2.6, now shows the deficiency of small nearest neighbour distances which is typical of regular patterns. For the Clark–Evans test, the observed value of $\bar{y}$ is 0.1283, the corresponding standard Normal deviate 6.30, and the conclusion emphatic rejection of CSR in favour of a regular alternative.

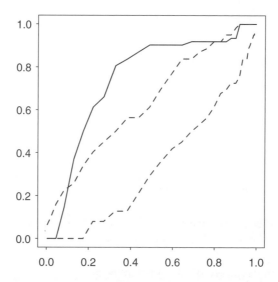

Figure 2.5. EDF plot of nearest neighbour distances for redwood seedlings: data (solid curve); upper and lower envelopes from 99 simulations of CSR (dashed curves).

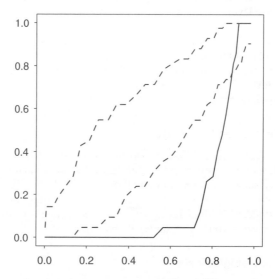

Figure 2.6. EDF plot of nearest neighbour distances for biological cells: data (solid curve); upper and lower envelopes from 99 simulations of CSR (dashed curves).

2.4 Point-to-nearest-event distances

A related type of analysis uses distances x_i from each of m sample points in A to the nearest of the n events. The EDF $\hat{F}(x) = m^{-1}\#(x_i \leq x)$ measures the empty spaces in A, in the sense that $1 - \hat{F}(x)$ is an estimate of the area $|B(x)|$ of the region $B(x)$ consisting of all points in A a distance at least x from every one of the n events in A. The argument leading to (2.9) can be repeated to show that, under CSR,

$$F(x) = 1 - \exp(-\pi\lambda x^2) : x \geq 0 \qquad (2.13)$$

approximately, where $\lambda = n|A|^{-1}$.

Lotwick (1981) describes an algorithm, based on the Green–Sibson Dirichlet tessellation algorithm, for computing $|B(x)|$ exactly when A is a rectangle. In practice, using m points in a regular $k \times k$ grid gives an adequate approximation if k is reasonably large. A sensible choice for k depends to some extent on the precise configuration of the n events in A and on the subsequent use to which the estimator will be put. Diggle and Matérn (1981) recommend $k \approx \sqrt{n}$ for estimating an unknown $F(x)$ from simulated realizations of a point process, in which context we have the freedom to choose both the number of sample points per realization and the number of realizations. Figure 2.7 shows, for the biological cells data, the degree of approximation introduced by using $k = 7 \approx \sqrt{42}$ or $k = 14$. In a modern computing context, concern about the computational effort of calculating $\hat{F}(x)$ is unnecessary, and there is certainly no good statistical reason to limit the choice of k. However, it is worth remembering that whilst large k will produce a very smooth curve $\hat{F}(x)$, its statistical precision is still limited by n, the number of events.

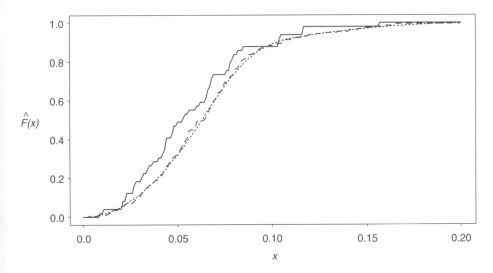

Figure 2.7. Calculation of $\hat{F}(x)$ for the biological cells data, using a $k \times k$ grid of sample points for different values of k: $k = 7$ (solid curve); $k = 14$ (dashed curve); $k = 96$ (dotted curve).

22 Statistical analysis of spatial point patterns

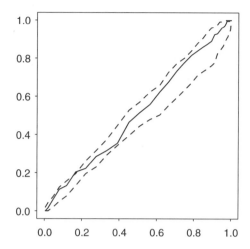

Figure 2.8. EDF plot of point-to-nearest-event distances for Japanese black pine saplings: data (solid curve); upper and lower envelopes from 99 simulations of CSR (dashed curves).

By analogy with the procedure adopted for nearest neighbour distances, a Monte Carlo test of CSR can be based on the statistic

$$u_i = \int \{\hat{F}_i(x) - \bar{F}_i(x)\}^2 \, dx. \tag{2.14}$$

2.4.1 Analysis of Japanese black pine saplings

Figure 2.8 shows the EDF plot for a point-to-nearest-event analysis of Numata's data, using $k=16$. We see that $\hat{F}_1(x)$ lies between the simulation envelopes and close to $\bar{F}_1(x)$ throughout its range. As in our previous analyses of these data, CSR is accepted.

2.4.2 Analysis of redwood seedlings

Figure 2.9 shows the corresponding EDF plot for the redwood data, again using $k=16$. Now $\hat{F}_1(x)$ lies below the lower simulation envelope for most of its range, and (2.14) leads to rejection of CSR with u_1 larger than all 99 simulated u_j. Note that $\hat{F}_1(x)$ drifts below the lower simulation envelope. This is typical of an aggregated pattern, and contrasts with the behaviour of $\hat{G}_1(y)$ for these data shown in Figure 2.5.

2.4.3 Analysis of biological cells

Figure 2.10 shows the comparable analysis of the biological cells, using $k=14$. A test based on (2.14) again leads to rejection of CSR with an attained significance level of 0.02. The position of $\hat{F}_1(x)$ near or above the upper simulation envelope typifies a regular pattern and again contrasts with the behaviour of $\hat{G}_1(y)$ for these data in Figure 2.6.

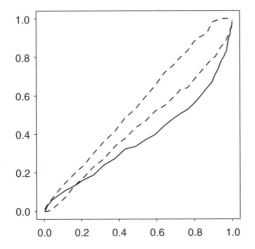

Figure 2.9. EDF plot of point-to-nearest-event distances for redwood seedlings: data (solid curve); upper and lower envelopes from 99 simulations of CSR (dashed curves).

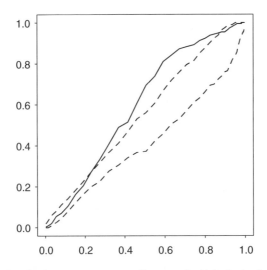

Figure 2.10. EDF plot of point-to-nearest-event distances for biological cells: data (solid curve); upper and lower envelopes from 99 simulations of CSR (dashed curves).

2.5 Quadrat counts

An alternative to a distance-based approach is to partition A into m sub-regions, or quadrats, of equal area and use the counts of numbers of events in the m quadrats to test CSR. The choice of sub-regions for this exercise is somewhat arbitrary. For ease of presentation, and because it represents common practice, we shall assume that A is the unit square and is partitioned into a regular $k \times k$ grid of square sub-regions, so that

24   Statistical analysis of spatial point patterns

$m=k^2$. Let $n_i : i=1,...,m$ be the quadrat counts which result from this partitioning of A and write $\bar{n}=n/m$ for the sample mean of the n_i. An obvious statistic to test for departures from the uniform distribution on A implied by CSR is Pearson's criterion,

$$X^2 = \sum_{i=1}^{m} (n_i - \bar{n})^2/\bar{n} \qquad (2.15)$$

whose null distribution is χ^2_{m-1}, to a good approximation provided that $\bar{n}$ is not too small.

Note that X^2 is just $m-1$ times the sample variance-to-mean ratio of the observed quadrat counts, which Fisher *et al.* (1922) introduced in order to test the hypothesis that the counts follow a Poisson distribution. The relationship between a uniform distribution of events and a Poisson distribution of quadrat counts is not entirely transparent, but is implicit in our definition of CSR and will be discussed further in Chapter 4. Note also that in the present context the null hypothesis may fail either because of a non-uniform distribution of events in A or because of dependencies amongst the events. In particular, significantly large or small values of X^2 are both of interest, and respectively indicate a tendency towards an aggregated or a regular spatial distribution of events in A.

2.5.1 Analysis of Japanese black pine saplings

For the 65 Japanese black pine saplings, the conservative rule that expected frequencies should be at least five suggests using a 3×3 grid. This gives an array of counts

$$\begin{array}{ccc} 6 & 15 & 7 \\ 10 & 4 & 3 \\ 4 & 8 & 8 \end{array}$$

for which $X^2 = 15.17$, corresponding to a one-sided attained significance level of $p = P(\chi^2_8 > 15.17) \approx 0.06$. Remembering that in the present context the chi-squared test is naturally two-sided, the evidence against CSR is weak; further support for this conclusion is provided by the fact that for both 4×4 and 2×2 grids the observed value of X^2 is close to its expectation under CSR.

2.5.2 Analysis of redwood seedlings

For the 62 redwood seedlings a 3×3 grid is again a reasonable choice. The observed counts are

$$\begin{array}{ccc} 5 & 9 & 6 \\ 13 & 8 & 2 \\ 0 & 6 & 13 \end{array}$$

and the X^2 value of 22.77 is highly significant ($p=0.0037$). A 4×4 grid similarly leads to emphatic rejection of CSR ($p=0.0010$), whereas a 2×2 grid gives $p=0.156$. A plausible model for these data, which we investigate further in Chapter 5, involves randomly distributed clusters of events and in these circumstances it is not unreasonable that the smaller-sized quadrats give the more emphatic rejection of CSR. The essential

Preliminary testing

point to note here is that the choice of quadrat size can have a marked effect on the result of the test.

2.5.3 Analysis of biological cells

For the 42 biological cells, the observed values of X^2 are below expectation for 2×2, 3×3 and 4×4 grids, significantly so in the 2×2 and 4×4 cases, although for a 4×4 grid the expected frequencies under CSR are a little small for comfort. The failure to reject CSR using the 3×3 grid suggests that the test is weak against regular alternatives to CSR. For comparison with the previous two examples, we give the 3×3 array of counts,

$$\begin{array}{ccc} 3 & 6 & 3 \\ 4 & 7 & 6 \\ 3 & 6 & 4 \end{array}$$

2.6 Scales of pattern

Greig-Smith (1952) proposed the following method for the analysis of data presented as counts in a large grid of contiguous quadrats. The sample variance-to-mean ratio, also called the index of dispersion, of the counts is first calculated for the basic grid and for further grids obtained by successive combination of adjacent quadrats into 2×2, 4×4, etc., *blocks*. The index of dispersion is then plotted against block size and peaks or troughs in the graph are interpreted as evidence of *scales of pattern* (aggregated or regular, respectively).

This method of analysis originated in plant ecology, in which field it became extremely popular; a review by Greig-Smith (1979) lists numerous applications. A possible objection to the method is that formal tests for the significance of peaks and troughs in the sequence of indices of dispersion at different scales are not available. According to the development in Section 2.5, each index is proportional to a chi-squared statistic for testing the hypothesis that the events are an independent random sample from the uniform distribution over the study region. Either this hypothesis is true or it is false – it makes no sense to ask whether it is true at some scales and false at others.

Mead (1974) addressed this formal defect of the Greig-Smith procedure by establishing a series of independent tests for pattern at several scales. Mead's procedure requires the data to be partitioned successively into 1, 4, 16, etc., blocks each consisting of 16 counts in a 4×4 grid. At each stage, the hypothesis to be tested is that, within each block, the set of counts in the four associated 2×2 sub-blocks is a random selection from $(16!)/(4!)^5 = 2\,627\,625$ equally likely possibilities, as implied by CSR. Mead's suggested test statistic is the sum of the six absolute pairwise differences between the four sub-block counts within a block, summed in turn over all blocks. A significantly large value of this statistic implies that, within blocks, counts in neighbouring quadrats are relatively similar, and this would be interpreted as evidence of aggregation at the appropriate scale. A significantly small value similarly implies relatively dissimilar counts in neighbouring quadrats. This is more difficult to interpret. An extreme manifestation of it would be a chess-board pattern of alternating high and low counts, but this seems unlikely to arise in practice. Once the test statistic, u say, has been chosen, the test itself can be implemented via Monte Carlo sampling of the null randomization distribution of u. The independence of the tests at the various scales

26 Statistical analysis of spatial point patterns

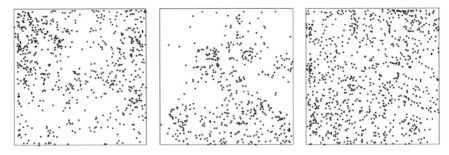

Figure 2.11. Locations of trees in Lansing woods: (left) hickories; (middle) maples; (right) oaks.

follows because the randomized 2×2 sub-block counts at one scale become the fixed 4×4 block counts at the next smaller scale, and so on.

So far, we have assumed that the quadrat grid has been superimposed retrospectively on a mapped pattern. In practice, the counts may be recorded directly in the field and a common variation, proposed by Kershaw (1957), is to replace the $k \times k$ grid by an $m \times 1$ transect. The data are then being analysed essentially as a time series, an analogy which is strengthened by Ripley's (1978) interpretation of Greig-Smith's method as a form of spectral analysis on the quadrat counts. By applying Greig-Smith's, Mead's and related methods to simulated data, Ripley also shows that the results can be difficult to interpret in terms of an underlying generating mechanism. From a modern statistical perspective, this is of greater concern than the lack of formal tests of significance.

2.6.1 Analysis of Lansing Woods data

Gerrard (1969) describes an investigation of a 19.6 acre square plot in Lansing Woods, Clinton County, Michigan, USA. In particular, he has provided the locations of 2251 trees in the plot. Maps of these data are shown, for the three major species groupings of hickories, maples and oaks, in Figure 2.11. Each map is here converted to counts in a 32×32 grid, which permits the investigation of four scales of pattern using Mead's procedure. The tests are implemented with 99 Monte Carlo randomizations, and the test statistic at each scale is the one suggested by Mead.

Table 2.1 gives the ranks of the observed test statistics amongst the Monte Carlo randomizations. For each of the three species groupings there is moderate or strong evidence of aggregation at the smallest scale and a strong indication of aggregation at one or more further scales. In the cases of the hickories and maples, departure from CSR is obvious from inspection of the data, but for the oaks the visual impression is much less clear. Figure 2.12 shows a plot of the quadrat count index of dispersion against block size, for each of the three species groupings. The sequence of generally increasing values of the index observed in each case is consistent with an underlying mechanism involving random variation in the local intensity of events, and in Chapters 7 and 8 we shall re-examine the data from this viewpoint. The plots in Figure 2.12 do not relate in any obvious way to the results of the analysis by Mead's procedure. This inconsistency was experienced also by Ripley (1978). It cannot be dismissed as an artefact of the Monte Carlo testing, but rather implies that the concept of a scale of pattern is somewhat ill-defined.

Table 2.1. Analysis of Lansing Woods data by Mead's procedure, using a 32 × 32 grid of quadrat counts and 99 randomizations: rank of u_1 amongst $u_i: i = 1, \ldots, 100$. A high rank for u_1 suggests aggregation. Where ties occur, the least extreme rank is quoted. Block size refers to the number of quadrats which are treated as a single 4 × 4 block

Species	Block size			
	4 × 4	8 × 8	16 × 16	32 × 32
Hickories	99	100	100	90
Maples	100	71	100	62
Oaks	95	99	90	73

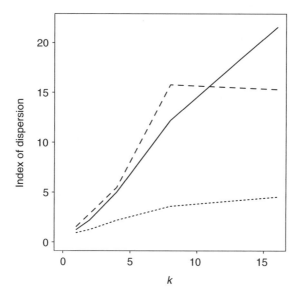

Figure 2.12. Index of dispersion plotted against block size ($k \times k$) for Lansing Woods data, based on a 32 × 32 grid of quadrat counts: hickories (solid curve); maples (dashed curve); oaks (dotted curve).

2.6.2 Scales of dependence

Besag (1978) describes a bivariate analogue of Mead's test in order to investigate what we might term *scales of dependence* between two patterns. For this, the basic unit is a 2 × 2 block of quadrats. Each quadrat provides a pair of counts, one for each species. Besag suggests testing the hypothesis that the two sets of four counts within a block are independent, using as test statistic the Spearman rank correlation coefficient (Kendall, 1970; Sprent, 1981, Chapter 10) for the two sets of four, summed over all blocks. The test is implemented via Monte Carlo randomization of counts within blocks. Each 2 × 2 block is then aggregated into a single quadrat, and so on, to give a sequence of independent tests of the hypothesis of independence for the two sets of counts within blocks. Besag applies this procedure to the Lansing Woods data and detects negative dependence between the hickories and maples, at the single scale corresponding to a partitioning of the study region into a 4 × 4 grid of blocks, i.e. an 8 × 8 grid of quadrats. The analysis of patterns formed by two or more distinct types of event will be considered in more detail in later chapters.

As noted in Section 1.2, contiguous quadrat counts represent a form of data intermediate between complete mapping and the sparse sampling procedures which we shall discuss in Chapter 3. Greig-Smith (1979) and Mead (1974) have emphasized that their analyses are intended to be exploratory in nature. As such, they are most useful for large, potentially heterogeneous data-sets, particularly if the results suggest further, and quite possibly non-statistical, investigations of the underlying processes.

2.7 Recommendations

The discussion in this chapter falls short of any systematic investigation of the power of the various tests under consideration. During the early development of the subject, many publications focused on tests of CSR and a number included comparative power assessments; see, for example, Ripley and Silverman (1978), Diggle (1979) and Ripley (1979a). Our recommendations are based partly on a synthesis of published results, but also on accumulated empirical experience.

Our overriding view is that a test of CSR is of very limited inherent interest, but rather should be seen as a framework within which exploratory analysis can be conducted. In our view, the most useful procedures are those based on functional summary descriptions of the data together with simulation envelopes to indicate the range of statistical variation under CSR. Of the three functional summaries considered in this chapter, we recommend using both $\hat{F}(\cdot)$ and $\hat{G}(\cdot)$ routinely. The two corresponding theoretical distribution functions, $F(\cdot)$ and $G(\cdot)$, are equal if the underlying point process is a homogeneous Poisson process, i.e. if CSR prevails, and departures from CSR typically induce opposite deviations in $\hat{F}(\cdot)$ and $\hat{G}(\cdot)$ from their common theoretical form under CSR. These deviations show up in the main body of each distribution, and are therefore easily seen from their graphical representations as EDF plots. For these reasons, it may be useful to combine the two types of nearest neighbour distance into a single test statistic. A possible test statistic, analogous to those used in Sections 2.3 and 2.4, would be

$$u_1 = \int \{\hat{F}(x) - \hat{G}(x)\}^2 \, dx$$

Another, suggested by Van Lieshout and Baddeley (1996), would be a statistic based on an estimate of the function $J(x) = \{1 - G(x)\}/\{1 - F(x)\}$. In this case, it is not necessary to use edge-corrected estimators for $F(\cdot)$ and $G(\cdot)$, as Van Lieshout and Baddeley have shown that the estimate of $J(\cdot)$ is insensitive to edge effects.

The functions $\hat{F}(\cdot)$ and $\hat{G}(\cdot)$, either separately or in combination, are also useful for assessing the goodness of fit to any other stochastic model. One reason for this is that they are complementary to the second-order methods and likelihood-based methods which, as we shall see in later chapters, are used in the initial formulation of models and in parameter estimation.

The inter-event distance distribution function, $H(\cdot)$, is less useful for preliminary testing. Its behaviour in our three illustrative examples, in which only the lower tail of the distribution is sensitive to quite pronounced changes in the underlying pattern, is typical. However, the distribution of inter-event distances is closely related to the second-order moment properties of a spatial point process and, as we shall see in later chapters, in this form it is a valuable tool in the much wider context of formulating and fitting stochastic models.

Quadrat count methods are now used infrequently for the analysis of mapped data. By comparison with the distance-based methods, they are less easily adaptable to more ambitious tasks, such as parameter estimation within a declared class of stochastic models.

3
Statistical methods for sparsely sampled patterns

3.1 General remarks

In this chapter we consider methods for the analysis of data obtained by a sparse sampling procedure, as defined in Section 1.2. We recall that such data consist either of *quadrat counts* in small areas within a study region A, or of distances measured from sampling points in A to neighbouring events. The number n of events in A is unknown, but must be assumed to be very much larger than m, the number of quadrats or sampling points, otherwise a complete mapping of A would presumably be feasible and would certainly be more informative. Typically, A will be large and potentially heterogeneous. For example, sparse sampling methods were originally devised for use in forestry surveys.

The objectives of a sparse sampling analysis will usually be to estimate the number of events in A, or equivalently the *intensity*, defined to be the mean number of events per unit area, and to obtain a qualitative description of the underlying pattern through the application of one or more tests of complete spatial randomness. If more detailed inferences are required, these are better dealt with by the collection and analysis of mapped data in sub-regions of A. Indeed, one useful function of a preliminary, sparse sampling analysis is to provide guidelines for the planning of a subsequent more detailed investigation.

Most theoretical discussions of sparse sampling assume, if only implicitly, that sample points are randomly located according to a uniform distribution on A. However, the essential practical requirement for the validity of the associated statistical methods is that sample points should be well separated in order that observations from different points can be assumed to be independent. This is most easily achieved by a systematic sampling design. Another desirable feature of systematic sampling is that it conveniently allows for retrospective partitioning of A into several sub-regions within which separate analyses can be performed and the results compared. A possible disadvantage is that the interval between successive sample points may coincide with periodicities in the underlying pattern. If this is thought to be a serious danger, it can be alleviated by random sampling within sub-regions of A. Other possible designs include, for example, the location of sample points along line transects. Note that the statistical merits of different sampling schemes should be compared on the basis of equal effort in the field. In this respect, systematic sampling may permit a larger value of m and, all other things being equal, a more sensitive analysis. In theory, the maximum value of m is constrained by the requirement that different sample points should generate independent observations. In practice, this constraint is not severe if systematic sampling is used. Byth and Ripley (1980) use simulations to establish that for any of the commonly used distance measurements, m may be at least as large as $0.1n$. If random sampling is used a safe upper limit is about $0.05n$. In the remainder of this chapter we assume without further comment that observations from different sample points are independent. Whatever sampling design is adopted, objectivity in the positioning of the sample points is vital in order to avoid biasing the subsequent quadrat counts or distance measurements.

In the remainder of this chapter, we first discuss separately the use of quadrat counts and distance methods for testing CSR and for estimating intensity. We then describe tests of independence between pairs of patterns, which are relevant to the interpretation of data like the Lansing Woods data in which different species are recorded within the same study region.

3.2 Quadrat counts

We recall from Section 1.4 that, under CSR, the number $N(B)$ of events in any region with area B follows a Poisson distribution with mean λB, where λ is the intensity. Explicitly, the probability distribution of $N(B)$ is

$$p_n(B) = \exp(-\lambda B)\{(\lambda B)^n/n!\} : n = 0, 1, 2, \ldots. \qquad (3.1)$$

In this section, we assume that the available data comprise independent counts $n_1, n_2, \ldots, n_m$ in m such quadrats, each of area B.

3.2.1 Tests of CSR

We wish to test the hypothesis that the n_i are an independent random sample from a Poisson distribution with unspecified mean. A natural test statistic is the sample variance-to-mean ratio or *index of dispersion*,

$$I = \sum_{i=1}^{m}(n_i - \bar{n})^2/\{(m-1)\bar{n}\}, \qquad (3.2)$$

whose intuitive appeal rests on the equality of the mean and variance of the Poisson distribution (3.1). Thus, I can be interpreted as a variance ratio statistic. The numerator,

$$s^2 = (m-1)^{-1}\sum_{i=1}^{m}(n_i - \bar{n})^2,$$

estimates the variance of $N(B)$ when no distributional assumptions are made, whilst the denominator, $\bar{n}$, estimates the variance when CSR holds. The index of dispersion was first used by Fisher *et al.* (1922). Under CSR, the sampling distribution of $(m-1)I$ is χ^2_{m-1}, to a good approximation provided that $m > 6$ and $\lambda B > 1$ (Kathirgamatamby, 1953). Significantly large or small values respectively indicate aggregated or regular departures from CSR. In Section 2.5 we showed that $(m-1)I$ could also be interpreted as Pearson's goodness-of-fit criterion for a uniform distribution of events over the union of the m quadrats, conditional on the total count.

32 Statistical analysis of spatial point patterns

The power of the index of dispersion test obviously increases with m, but also depends in an unpredictable way on the size and shape of the individual quadrats. Perry and Mead (1979) calculate the power of the test against a heterogeneous alternative to CSR involving interspersed patches of high and low intensity. Stiteler and Patil (1971) calculate the theoretical variance-to-mean ratio for some regular lattice patterns. Results in the above two papers and in Diggle (1979) suggest that the index of dispersion test is generally powerful against aggregated alternatives to CSR, but may be weak against regularity.

For quadrat count data, the index of dispersion appears to have no serious rivals as a test statistic. Cormack (1979) notes that alternative indices proposed by Morisita (1959) and by Lloyd (1967) need to be converted to $(m-1)I$ in order to test CSR.

Early work on the analysis of quadrat count data concentrated on the development of more general families of discrete distributions than the single-parameter Poisson, especially with a view to modelling aggregated patterns. See, for example, Evans (1953) or Douglas (1979). The story of the rise and fall of these so-called 'contagious distributions' as tools for the analysis of spatial data is of some historical interest because it shows how attempts to model observed data through discrete *distributions* ultimately foundered on their failure to respect the underlying setting of spatial point *processes*. We shall return to this in Chapter 5, as part of a wider discussion of the various classes of models which have been proposed for aggregated patterns.

3.2.2 Estimators of intensity

An intuitively reasonable estimator of the intensity is the total count divided by the total quadrat area,

$$\hat{\lambda} = \sum_{i=1}^{m} n_i/(mB). \tag{3.3}$$

It is easy to establish from (3.1) that this is the maximum likelihood estimator under CSR, in which case λ is unbiased for $\hat{\lambda}$, with variance $\lambda/(mB)$. More generally, $\hat{\lambda}$ is always an unbiased estimator for the intensity but its variance may depend on the size and shape of the individual quadrats and on the sampling scheme, as well as on the total quadrat area. Note that, strictly, the variance of $\hat{\lambda}$ is different according to whether it is regarded as an estimator for the observed number of events per unit area within A or for the intensity of an underlying spatial point process which is assumed to have generated the observed pattern: in the former case the variance goes to zero as a systematic sample of quadrats extends to cover the whole of A. In practice, the assumed sparseness of the sampling makes this distinction unimportant and the sample standard deviation of the observed counts can be used to construct interval estimates of λ. Some authors, including Ghent (1963), have suggested that in practice $\hat{\lambda}$ may be biased by a tendency for the field-worker to include events just outside the individual quadrat boundaries, in the mistaken belief that an empty quadrat contains no information.

3.2.3 Analysis of Lansing Woods data

We now apply these techniques to the Lansing Woods data introduced in Section 2.6, taking a systematic sample of 25 square quadrats of side 0.05 arranged in a 5×5 grid. We emphasize that this analysis is purely illustrative, because analysing a mapped

Table 3.1. Quadrat count analysis of Lansing Woods data, using 25 square quadrats of side 0.05

Species	λ	I	$\hat{\lambda}/\lambda$	$SE(\hat{\lambda}/\lambda)$
Hickories	703	2.59	1.02	0.25
Maples	514	2.92	0.90	0.29
Oaks	929	1.22	1.03	0.15

pattern by sparse sampling methods is inefficient. Table 3.1 gives the results for the analysis of each of the three species groupings. For the hickories and maples, CSR is overwhelmingly rejected in favour of an aggregated alternative, whilst for the oaks CSR is accepted (the one-sided 5% and 1% critical values of I when $m = 25$ are 1.52 and 1.79, respectively). In all three cases, $\hat{\lambda}$ is within one empirical standard error of λ, which we take to be equal to n because A is the unit square.

In these analyses, the individual counts are typically small (average counts for hickories, maples and oaks were 1.80, 1.16 and 2.40, respectively) but the quadrats are nevertheless physically quite large, as 0.05 translates to about 46 feet (14 metres) in the field. We repeated the analysis using 100 quadrats of side 0.02 and found marginal evidence against CSR for the maples and the oaks, but none at all for the hickories. However, the null distribution theory is suspect in this case because of the small average counts.

These results are generally consistent with, but weaker than, those obtained in Section 2.6 using a grid of contiguous quadrats to partition the whole of the study region.

3.3 Distance methods

Distance methods, also known as plotless sampling techniques, were introduced because of the practical difficulties sometimes raised by quadrat sampling. An early reference is Cottam and Curtis (1949). It is straightforward to devise a large number of subtly different distance methods, each with its own distribution theory. Possibly for this reason, an extensive literature on distance methods developed throughout the 1950s, 1960s and 1970s. Most of the early work was concerned with the definition of various types of distance measurement and associated statistics to test CSR or to estimate intensity. Holgate (1965a) marked something of a departure in that he evaluated the power functions of several tests of CSR against theoretical alternatives, thus providing an objective basis for the choice of a method. Developments since 1965 tended to continue in this vein, investigating the power of tests of CSR (Holgate, 1965b; Besag and Gleaves, 1973; Brown and Holgate, 1974; Diggle et al., 1976; Cox and Lewis, 1976; Diggle, 1977b; Hines and O'Hara Hines, 1979; Byth and Ripley, 1980) or the robustness of estimators of intensity (Persson, 1971; Pollard, 1971; Holgate, 1972; Diggle, 1975, 1977a; Cox, 1976; Warren and Batcheler, 1979; Patil et al., 1979; Byth, 1982).

3.3.1 Distribution theory under CSR

When CSR holds, the distribution theory for the various distance methods can be derived from the Poisson distribution of quadrat counts together with the independence

34 Statistical analysis of spatial point patterns

of counts in disjoint regions. From (3.1), taking B to be the area πx^2 of a disc of radius x, we immediately deduce that the distribution function of the distance X from an arbitrary point (or event) to the nearest (other) event is

$$F(x) = 1 - \exp(-\pi \lambda x^2) : x \geq 0, \qquad (3.4)$$

a result previously given in (2.9) and (2.13). Notice that πX^2 follows an exponential distribution with parameter λ and $2\pi \lambda X^2$ is therefore distributed as χ_2^2.

Various other distance distributions associated with the Poisson process can be derived from (3.1) and the independence of numbers of events in disjoint regions. Let $X_{k,\theta}$ denote the distance from an arbitrary point or event to the kth nearest event within a sector of included angle $\theta \leq 2\pi$ and arbitrary orientation. Let $U_k = \frac{1}{2}\theta X_{k,\theta}^2$ and note that U_k is the area of a sector of included angle θ and radius $X_{k,\theta}$. Then

$$P(U_1 > u_1) = P\{N(u_1) = 0\} = e^{-\lambda u_1},$$

again using (3.1). Furthermore, for any $u_2 > u_1$,

$$P(U_2 > u_2 \mid U_1 = u_1) = P\{N(u_2 - u_1) = 0\} = \exp\{-\lambda(u_2 - u_1)\},$$

so that the conditional probability density function (pdf) of U_2, given $U_1 = u_i$, is $\lambda \exp(-\lambda(u_2 - u_1))\}$ and the joint pdf of (U_1, U_2) is

$$f_2(u_1, u_2) = \lambda^2 \exp(-\lambda u_2) : 0 < u_1 < u_2.$$

Essentially the same argument gives the joint pdf of $(U_1, \ldots, U_k)$ for any k as

$$f_k(u_1, \ldots, u_k) = \lambda^k \exp(-\lambda u_k) : 0 < u_1 < \cdots < u_k, \qquad (3.5)$$

a result due to Thompson (1956).

More intricate geometrical constructions can be handled similarly. For example, Cox and Lewis (1976) consider the joint distribution of random variables X and Y defined as the respective distances from an arbitrary point O to the nearest event, at P say, and from P to the nearest other event, Q. Then

$$P(Y > y \mid X = x) = P[N\{A(x, y)\} = 0],$$

where

$$A(x, y) = \pi y^2 - (\phi y^2 + \theta x^2 - xy \sin \phi) \qquad (3.6)$$

is the area of the shaded region in Figure 3.1, $\cos \phi = y/(2x)$ and $\theta + 2\phi = \pi$.

Notice in particular that P is *not* an arbitrary event; the selection procedure for P is biased in favour of the more isolated events in the population. Cox and Lewis further deduce from (3.6) that, conditional on $Y > 2X$, the random variable $4X^2/Y^2$ is uniformly distributed on $(0, 1)$. Cormack (1977) uses a strikingly simple geometrical argument to show that this holds for *any* underlying pattern. Briefly, for an arbitrary pattern of events, consider the ith event to be located at the centre of a disc of radius $x_i/2$, where x_i is the distance from the ith event to its nearest neighbour. These circles

Statistical methods for sparsely sampled patterns

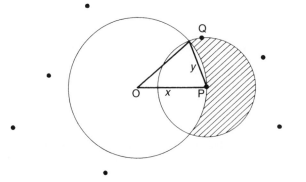

Figure 3.1. The nearest event to an arbitrary point.

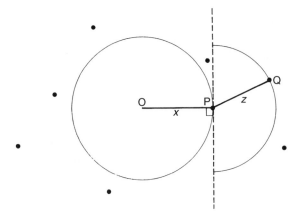

Figure 3.2. T-square sampling.

touch when pairs of events are reciprocal nearest neighbours, but cannot intersect. Conditioning on $Y > 2X$ is equivalent to placing the sampling origin O uniformly at random within the union of these discs, and the result follows.

A related, but distributionally simpler, device is the T-square sampling procedure of Besag and Gleaves (1973). As shown in Figure 3.2, O and P are as above, but Q is now the nearest event to P under the restriction that the angle OPQ must be at least $\pi/2$. With $X = \text{OP}$ as above and $Z = \text{PQ}$, we see that

$$P(Z > z | X = x) = P\{N(\pi z^2/2) = 0\} = \exp(-\lambda \pi x^2/2)$$

and deduce that $2\pi \lambda X^2$ and $\pi \lambda Z^2$ are independently and identically distributed as χ_2^2.

3.3.2 Tests of CSR

In this sub-section, remarks on the comparative power of different tests represent an overview of results in Diggle et al. (1976), Hines and O'Hara Hines (1979) and Byth and Ripley (1980). The original papers give more details in specific instances.

One general approach to the construction of a scale-free statistic to test CSR is to compare two types of distance measurement. For example, Hopkins (1954) considers measurements $x_i : i = 1, \ldots, m$ from each of m sample points to the nearest event and $y_i : i = 1, \ldots, m$ from each of m randomly sampled events to the nearest other event. Under CSR and sparse sampling, $2\pi\lambda x_i^2$ and $2\pi\lambda y_i^2$ are independently distributed as χ_2^2. Thus, $2\pi\lambda \sum_{i=1}^m x_i^2$ and $2\pi\lambda \sum_{i=1}^m y_i^2$ are independently distributed as χ_{2m}^2 and

$$h = \sum x_i^2 \Big/ \sum y_i^2 \tag{3.7}$$

is distributed as $F_{2m,2m}$. In (3.7), and in the remainder of this section unless stated otherwise, summations are over $i = 1, \ldots, m$. The rationale for Hopkins's test is that in an aggregated pattern, the point–event distances x_i will be large relative to the event–event distances y_i, and vice versa in a regular pattern. Thus, significantly large or small values of h indicate aggregation or regularity, respectively. Note that $h/(1 + h)$ lies between 0 and 1 and could be regarded as an index of pattern. The statistic h was proposed independently by Moore (1954).

Within the context of sparse sampling methods, Hopkins' test generally has good power properties. Unfortunately, however, the random selection of events requires a complete enumeration within A, which is precisely the operation we wish to avoid in a sparse sampling analysis. Byth and Ripley (1980) propose implementing Hopkins' test, but selecting one event at random from each of m quadrats 'of a size which would contain about five trees on average'. In some contexts this might still prove impractical, and would in any case imply an increased effort in the field which has not been allowed for in published power comparisons.

Holgate (1965b) considers measurements $(x_{1i}, x_{2i}) : i = 1, \ldots, m$ from each of m sample points to the nearest and second nearest events, respectively. He then uses (3.5) to deduce that, under CSR, x_{1i}^2/x_{2i}^2 is uniformly distributed on $(0, 1)$, whence

$$h_N = m^{-1} \sum \left(x_{1i}^2/x_{2i}^2\right)$$

is Normally distributed with mean 1 and variance $(12m)^{-1}$, to an excellent approximation if $m > 10$. Alternatively,

$$h_F = \sum x_{1i}^2 \Big/ \sum \left(x_{2i}^2 - x_{1i}^2\right)$$

is distributed as $F_{2m,2m}$. The rationale for h_F is that $(x_{2i}^2 - x_{1i}^2)$ should behave like y_i^2, and the interpretation of h_N or h_F is the same as for Hopkins's h. Published results suggest that Holgate's tests are generally less powerful than Hopkins's test and, in particular, are very weak against regular alternatives to CSR.

Eberhardt (1967) considered only point–event distances x_i, and proposed an index

$$e = m \sum x_i^2 \Big/ \left(\sum x_i\right)^2.$$

Note that $\sqrt{\{m(e-1)/(m-1)\}}$ is the sample coefficient of variation of the distances x_i. Hines and O'Hara Hines (1979) provide critical values to test CSR but the test must be weak against aggregated alternatives, because the distribution of e under CSR applies also to a process of randomly distributed point clusters, in which each single event of a completely random pattern is replaced by a fixed or random number of coincident events. By the same argument, any scale-free statistic based only on measurements of the distance from a sample point to the nearest event must be suspect.

Besag and Gleaves (1973) use data $(x_i, z_i) : i = 1, \ldots, m$ generated by their T-square sampling procedure as described in Section 3.3.1; recall that x_i is a point–event distance and z_i an event–event distance in a restricted area of search. Two possible test statistics are

$$t_N = m^{-1} \sum x_i^2 / (x_i^2 + z_i^2/2) \tag{3.8}$$

and

$$t_F = 2 \sum x_i^2 / \sum z_i^2,$$

whose distributions under CSR are the same as for the corresponding Holgate statistics h_N and h_F. Significantly large or small values again suggest aggregation or regularity, respectively. The T-square tests are generally less powerful than Hopkins's test but more powerful than their Holgate counterparts, particularly against regular alternatives. On balance, t_N is preferable to t_F, although this does depend on the range of alternatives under consideration. Hines and O'Hara Hines (1979) recommend a variant of Eberhardt's index based on T-square sampling. In this variant, the measurements x_i and $z_i/\sqrt{2}$, which under CSR are independent with a common distribution given by (3.4), are treated as a single sample of size $2m$. The resulting test statistic appears to be slightly more powerful than t_N against a range of aggregated and regular alternatives, although its interpretation is less transparent.

One advantage of the T-square sampling procedure is that the simplicity of its distribution theory under CSR allows to some extent for the development of appropriate tests when the range of alternatives is restricted a priori. For example, a test based on t_N is insensitive to long-range fluctuations in local intensity. Specifically, if CSR applies locally but with possibly different values, λ_i say, of the intensity parameter associated with the m sample points, the distribution of t_N is the same as under CSR. However, within this restricted context it is straightforward to derive the likelihood ratio test of CSR, which corresponds to equal λ_i. The test statistic is

$$M = 48m \left\{ m \log(\bar{u}) - \sum \log u_i \right\} / (13m + 1), \tag{3.9}$$

where $u_i = x_i^2 + z_i^2/2$. The approximate distribution of M under CSR is χ^2_{m-1}. This test is a direct analogue of Bartlett's (1937) test of the equality of variances in Normal sampling and incorporates the correction factor recommended by Bartlett to improve the chi-squared approximation. Note that the test is one-sided: significantly large values suggest rejection of CSR. Diggle (1977b) proposed a two-stage procedure in which the M-test is applied only if an initial test using t_N gives a non-significant result. The effect of this is to achieve a four-way classification of the underlying pattern as regular, random, heterogeneous or aggregated, although the two-stage procedure means that the nominal significance level for M is not strictly correct.

Another situation in which the standard tests are unsatisfactory is when elements of aggregation and regularity are combined. For example, Brown and Rothery (1978) discuss the detection of local regularity in the presence of long-range aggregation, motivated by a study of the spacing of ducks' nests when only a small proportion of

38 Statistical analysis of spatial point patterns

the study region contains usable nesting sites (Brown, 1975). In this context, T-square sampling will typically generate point–event distances x_i which are larger than the event–event distances z_i, indicating aggregation. The local regularity could be detected by using only the z_i; two possible statistics are the Eberhardt index or a variant of the M statistic,

$$M = 24m \left\{ m \log(\overline{z^2}) - \sum \log z_i^2 \right\} \Big/ (7m+1),$$

with significantly *small* values of either statistic indicating regularity.

Cox and Lewis (1976) work with data $(x_i, y_i) : i = 1, \ldots, m$, where x_i is the distance from the ith sample point to the nearest event and y_i the distance from that event to the nearest other event. As described in Section 3.3.1 above, Cormack (1977) shows that pairs (x_i, y_i) with $y_i > 2x_i$ are uninformative. Cox and Lewis consider the $m_0 \leq m$ pairs for which $y_i < 2x_i$, and use (3.6) to show that the following sequence of transformations produces observations $r_i : i = 1, \ldots, m$, whose distribution under CSR is uniform on $(0, 1)$:

(i) $\theta_i = 2\sin^{-1}\{y_i/(2x_i)\}$;
(ii) $w_i = \{2\pi + \sin\theta_i - (\pi + \theta_i)\cos\theta_i\}^{-1}$;
(iii) $r_i = (4\pi w_i - 1)/3$.

Thus, $cl = m_0^{-1} \sum_{i=1}^{m_0} r_i$ is approximately Normally distributed with mean 0.5 and variance $(12m_0)^{-1}$ under CSR. Significantly large or small values indicate aggregation or regularity respectively, and in either case the power of the test appears to be comparable to that of t_N.

An ingenious sampling procedure whose statistical potential appears not to have been tapped is Catana's (1963) 'wandering quarter'. This generates a single point–event distance x_0 and a sequence of event–event distances $x_i : i = 1, \ldots, m$ from a single starting point O, as indicated in Figure 3.3. Under CSR, the transformed observations πx_i^2 are independently distributed as χ_2^2. Inferential procedures could, and should, recognize the spatial ordering of the x_i. For example, the method could be used to sample a square region by a series of parallel traverses. Each traverse defines a one-dimensional spatial series, and simple plotting of each series with x_i as ordinate

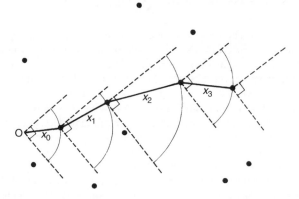

Figure 3.3. Catana's wandering quarter.

3.3.3 Estimators of intensity

Suppose now that distances are measured from each sample point to the nearest, second nearest, ... kth nearest event. Then (3.5) shows that under CSR the distances x_{ki} : $i = 1, \ldots, m$ to kth nearest events are sufficient for λ, and the maximum likelihood estimator of $\gamma = \lambda^{-1}$ is

$$\hat{\gamma}_k = \pi \left(\sum x_{ki}^2 \right) \Big/ (km)$$

which is unbiased with variance $\gamma^2/(km)$. An increase in the value of k gives an estimator which has smaller variance, but whose application in the field is more time-consuming. The more subtle question of robustness to departures from CSR will be considered shortly. The change from λ to γ as the parameter of interest makes for ease of presentation, but also seems natural for a distance-based method of estimation, since squared distances effectively measure areas. Holgate (1964) showed that if the total quadrat area in the quadrat count estimator (3.5) is set equal to the expected area of search involved in computing $\hat{\gamma}_k^{-1}$, considered as an estimator for λ, then the two methods are equally efficient under CSR and, incidentally, all choices of k in $\hat{\gamma}_k$ are equally efficient.

The major objection to $\hat{\gamma}_k$ is that it can be seriously biased when CSR does not hold (Persson, 1971; Pollard, 1971). The bias tends to become smaller for larger values of k, but identifying the kth nearest neighbour in the field then becomes difficult. An alternative strategy for reducing the bias is to note that estimators based on point–event and on event–event distances tend to be biased in opposite directions. An average of the two should therefore be more robust, in the sense of having smaller bias for a wide range of underlying patterns. Under CSR, the maximum likelihood estimator for γ based on a T-square sample $(x_i, z_i) : i = 1, \ldots, m$ is

$$\hat{\gamma}_T = \pi \left(\sum x_i^2 + \sum z_i^2/2 \right) \Big/ (2m),$$

the arithmetic mean of estimators based on the x_i or z_i measurements separately. Results in Diggle (1975, 1977a) suggest that a more robust estimator is

$$\gamma_T^* = (\pi/m) \sqrt{\left(2 \sum x_i^2 \Big/ \sum z_i^2 \right)},$$

whilst Byth (1982) recommends

$$\tilde{\gamma}_T = (2\sqrt{2}/m^2) \left(\sum x_i \sum z_i \right), \tag{3.10}$$

which is less sensitive than γ_T^* to an occasional very large x_i measurement in a strongly aggregated pattern.

Because $\tilde{\gamma}_T$ is a function of two sample means, its approximate standard error can be calculated using the delta technique. Let $\bar{x}, \bar{z}, s_x^2, s_z^2$ and s_{xz} denote sample means, variances and covariance. Then,

$$SE(\tilde{\gamma}_T) \approx \sqrt{\{8(\bar{z}^2 s_x^2 + 2\bar{x}\bar{z}s_{xz} + \bar{x}^2 s_z^2)/m\}}.$$

Table 3.2. T-square analysis of Lansing Woods data. Figures in parentheses indicate attained significance levels for tests of CSR (two-sided for t_N, one-sided for M)

Species	γ	t_N	M	$\tilde{\gamma}_T/\gamma$	$SE(\tilde{\gamma}_T/\gamma)$
Hickories	0.001425	0.54 (0.53)	41.26 (0.02)	1.47	0.26
Maples	0.001946	0.60 (0.08)	38.28 (0.03)	1.23	0.29
Oaks	0.001076	0.42 (0.17)	32.18 (0.12)	0.99	0.15

Strictly, this does not lead to interval estimates for γ but for $E(\tilde{\gamma}_T)$. However, it would appear that the bias of $\tilde{\gamma}_T$ is often small. It is admittedly easy to devise theoretical point process models for which $\tilde{\gamma}_T$ performs badly, but these typically represent extreme departures from CSR which would be easily detected in the field. One example would be a process involving large, tightly clustered groups of events, in which case it would be more sensible to estimate separately the mean area per cluster and the mean cluster size.

Cox (1976) and Warren and Batcheler (1979) adopt a different approach in which an empirically determined correction factor is applied to an estimator based only on point–event distances. Warren and Batcheler report a variety of successful applications, but Byth (1982) obtains disappointing results from a simulation study.

Patil et al. (1979) devise a consistent estimator for the intensity of any stationary process which does not generate multiple coincident events, but this theoretically desirable property appears to have been achieved at the expense of a large increase in variance.

3.3.4 Analysis of Lansing Woods data

We again use the Lansing Woods data to illustrate the use of sparse sampling techniques, in this case T-square sampling. We take a systematic sample of $m = 25$ points in a 5×5 grid. To test CSR we use the t_N statistic (3.8) followed if necessary by the M statistic (3.9). To estimate γ, the mean area per event, we use Byth's estimator $\tilde{\gamma}_T$, defined in (3.10). The results are given in Table 3.2. We accept CSR for the oaks, but reject CSR in favour of a heterogeneous alternative for both the hickories and the maples. The estimates of $\tilde{\gamma}_T$ are within one empirical standard error of γ except for the hickories, where the difference is about 1.8 standard errors.

3.4 Tests of independence

When events of two different types, for example plants of different species, co-exist within a study region, it may be of interest to establish whether the two underlying point processes are independent.

For quadrat count data, the hypothesis under test is that the two sets of counts are independent, but with unspecified marginal distributions. Because the data are discrete, they are naturally presented as a two-way table of frequencies and the hypothesis of independence, conditional on the marginal totals, can be tested via Pearson's X^2 statistic or its asymptotic equivalent, the likelihood ratio statistic for interaction between rows and columns in a Poisson log-linear model. Note that this does *not* assume that the counts are marginally Poisson-distributed.

For a distance-based approach, an early contribution was made by Goodall (1965) who observed that, under independence, the distances from an arbitrary point to the nearest type 2 event, and from an arbitrary type 1 event to the nearest type 2 event, would be independent and identically distributed. In this context, treating the nearest type 1 event to an arbitrary point as an arbitrary type 1 event would not invalidate a test of independence of the two types of event. It would affect the power of the test, as would switching the labelling of the two types. For example, consider a process in which type 1 events form a Poisson process and a proportion p of type 1 events have an associated type 2 event a small distance away. If p is small, the test as described will be weak, whereas interchanging the role of the two types of event would give a more powerful test since every type 2 event has an associated type 1 event close by, but not conversely.

Diggle and Cox (1981) propose as test statistic Kendall's rank correlation coefficient τ (Kendall, 1970; Sprent, 1981, Chapter 10) between pairs of distances from each of n sample points to the nearest events of type 1 and type 2. Their comparative simulations suggest that this test is more powerful than Goodall's test against a range of positively or negatively dependent alternatives to independence.

3.5 Recommendations

It is difficult to compare the statistical merits of quadrat count and distance methods because they are based on quite different sampling operations, and their relative ease of implementation in the field will vary considerably between applications.

For a quadrat count analysis, the choice of which statistic to use for testing or estimation is straightforward. In contrast, the choice of quadrat size is rather arbitrary and can seriously affect the results of the analysis. With this qualification, the index of dispersion (3.1) provides a test of CSR which is generally powerful against aggregation, but less so against regularity. The intensity estimator $\hat{\lambda}$ defined at (3.3) is always unbiased.

Amongst the many distance-based methods, T-square sampling is easy to use in the field, and the simplicity of its associated distribution theory gives some degree of flexibility in the construction of tests of CSR and estimators of intensity. To test CSR, the combination of t_N and M allows a four-way classification of the underlying pattern as regular, random, heterogeneous or aggregated, with good power against each type of alternative. To estimate the mean area per event, the estimator $\tilde{\gamma}_T$ is generally robust, although unbiasedness is not guaranteed.

Finally, note that sparse sampling methods are inherently limited in what they can achieve by comparison with methods for the analysis of mapped data. In this respect, we again emphasize that the current discussion of the Lansing Woods data is purely illustrative.

4
Spatial point processes

4.1 Processes and summary descriptions

A *spatial point process* is a stochastic mechanism which generates a countable set of events x_i in the plane. We will usually be dealing with processes which are *stationary* and *isotropic*. Stationarity means that all properties of the process are invariant under translation, isotropy that they are invariant under rotation. These assumptions are less restrictive than they might seem at first sight. In particular, they do not rule out the modelling of *random* heterogeneity in the environment (cf. the discussion of Figure 1.2 in Section 1.1). However, three qualifications are in order.

Firstly, although models are often defined as processes on the whole plane, in practice we only apply them to data from finite planar regions and it will be sufficient for our purposes if stationarity and isotropy hold to a reasonable approximation within the study region in question. Indeed, study regions are often selected with this requirement implicitly in mind so that, for example, in microanatomical studies the tissue sections to be analysed are deliberately sited well away from any boundaries between different types of tissue.

Secondly, we will abandon the stationarity assumption when the data include spatial explanatory variables which are thought to affect the local intensity of events.

Finally, in some applications we may choose to circumvent the stationarity assumption by the use of design-based inference. This applies to the analysis of replicated patterns as discussed in Chapter 8, and to certain problems in environmental epidemiology which we consider in Chapter 9.

Statistical methods for spatial point pattern data often involve comparisons between empirical summary descriptions of the data and the corresponding theoretical summary descriptions of a point process model. However, it is important that the theoretical summary descriptions are derived from an underlying model, rather than being advanced as models in their own right. For example, we have already seen in Chapter 2 that one summary description of the homogeneous Poisson process is that the distribution function of the distance from an arbitrary event of the process to its nearest neighbour is

$$G(y) = 1 - \exp(-\lambda \pi y^2) \; : \; y \geq 0.$$

This leads, amongst other things, to the construction of tests of CSR involving a comparison between this theoretical form of $G(y)$ and the corresponding empirical distribution function for an observed pattern of n events. However, it would make no sense to attempt to define a more general class of models by embedding $G(y)$ within a larger parametric family of distributions unless the enlarged class were itself derived from an explicit class of point process models.

In this chapter, we consider various theoretical summary descriptions of point processes, and the corresponding empirical descriptions of point pattern data. We focus on properties which lead to useful statistical methods, and illustrate their use on a number of data-sets. We include a description of the homogeneous Poisson process and, for multivariate processes, discuss the ideas of independence and random labelling. We postpone until Chapter 5 a general discussion of different parametric classes of point processes which have been proposed as models for data.

We need the following notation: $E[X]$ denotes the expectation of a random variable X; $N(A)$ denotes the number of events in the planar region A; in a multivariate process, $N_j(A)$ similarly denotes the number of type j events in A; $|A|$ is the area of A; dx is an infinitesimal region which contains the point x; $||x - y||$ denotes the Euclidean distance between the points x and y.

4.2 Second-order properties

4.2.1 Univariate processes

We can now define the *first-order* and *second-order* properties of a spatial point process. First-order properties are described by an *intensity function*,

$$\lambda(x) = \lim_{|dx| \to 0} \left\{ \frac{E[N(dx)]}{|dx|} \right\}.$$

For a stationary process, $\lambda(x)$ assumes a constant value λ, the mean number of events per unit area. The *second-order intensity function* is similarly defined as

$$\lambda_2(x, y) = \lim_{|dx|,|dy| \to 0} \left\{ \frac{E[N(dx)N(dy)]}{|dx||dy|} \right\}.$$

A closely related quantity is the *conditional intensity* $\lambda_c(x|y) = \lambda_2(x, y)/\lambda(y)$ which, loosely speaking, corresponds to the intensity at the point x conditional on the information that there is an event at y.

For a stationary process, $\lambda_2(x, y) \equiv \lambda_2(x - y)$; for a stationary, isotropic process, $\lambda_2(x - y)$ reduces further to $\lambda_2(t)$, where $t = ||x - y||$. In statistical mechanics, the scaled quantity $\lambda_2(t)/\lambda^2$ is referred to as the *radial distribution function*, although it is not a distribution function in the usual statistical sense.

Baddeley et al. (2000) discuss *reweighted (second-order) stationary* processes, which have the property that $\lambda_2(x, y)/\lambda(x)\lambda(y) = \rho(t)$ depends only on $t = ||x - y||$. Note that this requires $\lambda(\cdot)$ to be bounded away from zero. Reweighted stationarity is a point process analogue of the assumption commonly made in the analysis of real-valued spatial processes that the mean may vary spatially whereas the variation about the local mean is stationary.

An alternative characterization of the second-order properties of a stationary, isotropic process is provided by the function $K(t)$, one definition of which is

$$K(t) = \lambda^{-1} E[N_0(t)], \tag{4.1}$$

where $N_0(t)$ is the number of further events within distance t of an arbitrary event. The notion of an arbitrary event of the process involves the conceptual limit of simple random sampling from a finite population. For a mathematically rigorous discussion see, for example, Daley and Vere-Jones (1972). Intuitively, we envisage a large but finite number n of events in some finite region. An event selected at random from this population is, by definition, an arbitrary event. Similarly, in practice an arbitrary point will mean a point distributed uniformly over some finite region.

In order to establish a link between $K(t)$ and $\lambda_2(t)$ we shall assume that our process is *orderly*, by which we mean that multiple coincident events cannot occur or, more precisely, that $P\{N(dx) > 1\}$ is of a smaller order of magnitude than $|dx|$. This means that $E[N(dx)] \sim P\{N(dx) = 1\}$ in the sense that the ratio of these two quantities tends to 1 as $|dx| \to 0$. We shall further assume that in a similar sense, $E[N(dx)N(dy)] \sim P\{N(dx) = N(dy) = 1\}$. Under these conditions, the expected number of further events within distance t of an arbitrary event can be computed by integrating the conditional intensity over the disc with centre the origin, denoted 0, and radius t. Hence,

$$\lambda K(t) = \int_0^{2\pi} \int_0^t \{\lambda_c\}(x|o) x \, dx \, d\theta.$$

Using the fact that $\lambda_c(x|o) = \lambda_2(x)/\lambda$, this gives

$$\lambda K(t) = 2\pi \lambda^{-1} \int_0^t \lambda_2(x) x \, dx, \tag{4.2}$$

or conversely,

$$\lambda_2(t) = \lambda^2 (2\pi t)^{-1} K'(t). \tag{4.3}$$

Note that for a reweighted stationary process, Baddeley *et al.* (2000) extend the definition of the K-function to

$$K_I(t) = 2\pi \int_0^t \rho(x) x \, dx,$$

which reduces to (4.2) in the stationary case.

From a theoretical viewpoint it is sometimes more convenient to work with $\lambda_2(t)$ rather than with $K(t)$, and as a minor variation we define a *covariance density*,

$$\gamma(t) = \lambda_2(t) - \lambda^2. \tag{4.4}$$

For data analysis, one advantage of $K(t)$ over $\lambda_2(t)$ is that it can more easily be estimated automatically from a set of data. Essentially, $K(t)$ and $\lambda_2(t)$ are related to the distribution function and probability density function of the distances between pairs of events in a point pattern and, especially in small samples, it is convenient that the former can be estimated without having to decide how much to smooth the corresponding empirical distribution.

Another useful property of the K-function is that it is invariant under random thinning. By this, we mean that if each event of a process is retained or not according to a series of mutually independent Bernoulli trials, then the K-function of the resulting thinned process is identical to that of the original, unthinned process. This follows from the definition (4.1), where the K-function is defined as the ratio of two quantities,

$E[N_0(t)]$ and λ. The effect of the thinning is to multiply each of these by p, the retention probability for any one event, leaving the ratio unchanged.

Rather than observe the exact locations of events in a planar region, it is sometimes easier in practice to observe only counts $N(A)$ in convenient sub-regions A (cf. Section 2.6). The resulting *quadrat count distribution*,

$$p_n(A) = P\{N(A) = n\} \ : \ n = 0, 1, \ldots,$$

provides a possible summary description of the process. The arbitrary nature of A is unsatisfactory. One solution is further to summarize the quadrat count distribution by its first few moments, and to regard these as functions of A. In particular,

$$E[N(A)] = \int_A \lambda(x) dx,$$

which reduces to $\lambda |A|$ for a stationary process. More interestingly, orderliness implies that

$$E[N(A)^2] = E\left[\left\{\int_A N(dx)\right\}^2\right]$$
$$= E\left[\int_A N(dx) + \int_A \int_A N(dx)N(dy)\right].$$

Interchanging expectation and integration, this becomes, for a stationary process,

$$\lambda|A| + \int_A \int_A \lambda_2(x-y) dx\, dy,$$

whence

$$\text{Var}\{N(A)\} = \int_A \int_A \lambda_2(x-y) dx\, dy + \lambda|A|(1 - \lambda|A|). \tag{4.5}$$

A straightforward generalization gives

$$\text{Cov}\{N(A), N(B)\} = \int_A \int_B \lambda_2(x-y) dx\, dy + \lambda|A \cap B| - \lambda^2 |A||B|,$$

where $A \cap B$ denotes the intersection of A and B.

The quantity $\text{Var}\{N(A)\}$ defined in (4.5) is sometimes called the 'variance-area curve', and is closely related to $K(t)$ in the sense that both involve integrated versions of the second-order intensity function.

4.2.2 Extension to multivariate processes

In a *multivariate* process, the events are of two or more distinguishable types. Definitions for the second-order properties of such processes follow as natural generalizations of the corresponding quantities for univariate processes. We assume stationarity, isotropy and orderliness, and write $N_j(S)$ for the number of type j events in a planar region A.

The *(first-order) intensities* are constants,

$$\lambda_j = \mathrm{E}[N_j(A)]/|A|.$$

The *second-order intensities* are functions of a scalar argument,

$$\lambda_{ij}(t) = \lim_{\substack{|dx|\to 0 \\ |dy|\to 0}} \left\{ \frac{\mathrm{E}[N_i(dx)N_j(dy)]}{|dx||dy|} \right\}$$

where, as before, t denotes distance. The corresponding *covariance densities* are

$$\gamma_{ij}(t) = \lambda_{ij}(t) - \lambda_i \lambda_j$$

and the multivariate K-functions are

$$K_{ij}(t) = \lambda_j^{-1} \mathrm{E}[N_{0ij}(t)], \tag{4.6}$$

where $N_{0ij}(t)$ denotes the expected number of (further) type j events within distance t of an arbitrary type i event. Note that $\lambda_{ij}(t) = \lambda_{ji}(t)$, from which it follows that $\gamma_{ij}(t) = \gamma_{ji}(t)$. A similar argument to the one used in Section 4.2.1 shows that

$$K_{ij}(t) = 2\pi (\lambda_i \lambda_j)^{-1} \int \lambda_{ij}(x) x\, dx,$$

from which it follows that $K_{ji}(t) = K_{ij}(t)$.

4.3 Higher-order moments and nearest neighbour distributions

Second-order properties provide a natural and valuable starting point for the description of a spatial point process. However, they do not give a complete picture. Baddeley and Silverman (1984) describe a class of non-Poisson processes for which $K(t) = \pi t^2$, and in Section 5.8.3 we shall give another example in which clearly different processes have identical second-order properties. Higher-order properties can easily be defined in terms of the joint intensity functions for the occurrence of specified configurations of three, four, etc. events. Interpretation would be difficult in practice since, for example, the third-order intensity function of a stationary, isotropic process requires three arguments, the fourth-order function five, and so on.

In view of this, we define two distribution functions which were used in Chapter 2 to provide tests of CSR and which serve as additional summary descriptions for spatial point processes. These are $G(y)$, the distribution function of the distance from an arbitrary *event* to the nearest other event, and $F(x)$, the distribution function of the distance from an arbitrary *point* to the nearest event.

One interpretation of $F(x)$ is as the probability that a randomly located disc of radius x contains at least one event. This suggests an obvious extension whereby the disc is replaced by some other geometrical figure. Oriented shapes such as ellipses or rectangles could be used to describe departures from isotropy. Matheron (1975) incorporates these ideas within a general theory of random sets, in which a random set S is characterized by the function $\mathcal{F}(T)$, the probability that the intersection of S with T is non-empty, for each of a wide variety of 'test-sets' T.

4.4 The homogeneous Poisson process

The homogeneous planar Poisson process, subsequently referred to without qualification as the Poisson process, is the cornerstone on which the theory of spatial point processes is built. It represents the simplest possible stochastic mechanism for the generation of spatial point patterns, and in applications is used as an idealized standard of CSR which, if strictly unattainable in practice, sometimes provides a useful approximate description of an observed pattern. The Poisson process is conveniently defined by the following postulates, which correspond exactly to the definition of CSR given in Section 1.4:

PP1 For some $\lambda > 0$, and any finite planar region A, $N(A)$ follows a Poisson distribution with mean $\lambda |A|$.

PP2 Given $N(A) = n$, the n events in A form an independent random sample from the uniform distribution on A.

To demonstrate that PP1 and PP2 are self-consistent, we first establish:

PP3 For any two disjoint regions A and B, the random variables $N(A)$ and $N(B)$ are independent.

Let $C = A \cup B$ be the union of two disjoint regions A and B. Write $p = |A|/|C|$ and $q = 1 - p = |B|/|C|$. Then, PP2 applied to region C implies that

$$P\{N(A) = x, N(B) = y | N(C) = n\} = \binom{x+y}{x} p^x q^y,$$

for integers $0 \le x \le n$ and $y = n - x$. PP1 then gives the unconditional joint distribution of $N(A)$ and $N(B)$ as

$$P\{N(A) = x, N(B) = y\} = \binom{x+y}{x} p^x q^y \{e^{-\lambda|C|}(\lambda|C|)^n / n!\}$$

$$= \{e^{-\lambda|A|}(\lambda|A|)^x / x!\}\{e^{-\lambda|B|}(\lambda|B|)^y / y!\} \quad (4.7)$$

for all integers $x \ge 0$ and $y \ge 0$. This establishes PP3 and shows also that $N(A)$ and $N(B)$ have the distributions implied by PP1. It is immediately obvious that if PP2 holds for any region C it must hold also for all sub-regions of C. Conversely, the additive property of independent Poisson-distributed random variables X and Y, and the associated conditional binomial distribution of X given $X + Y$, establish PP1 and PP2 respectively for any region formed as the union of two disjoint regions for which PP1 and PP2 hold. This proves the required self-consistency.

The parameter λ of the Poisson process is its intensity. The independence result PP3 implies that

$$\lambda_2(t) = \lambda^2 \; : \; t > 0, \quad (4.8)$$

whence (4.2) gives

$$K(t) = \pi t^2 \; : \; t > 0. \quad (4.9)$$

The variance-area curve follows directly from PP1 as

$$\mathrm{Var}\{N(A)\} = \lambda|A|. \quad (4.10)$$

The nearest neighbour distribution functions $G(y)$ and $F(x)$ are identical, since the existence of an event at a particular point, x_0 say, has no bearing on the distribution of the remaining number of events in a disc with centre x_0. We deduce from PP1 that

$$F(x) = G(x) = P\{N(\pi x^2) > 0\} = 1 - \exp(-\pi \lambda x^2) \; : \; x > 0. \tag{4.11}$$

To simulate a partial realization of a Poisson process on A conditional on a fixed value of $N(A)$, we need to generate events independently according to a uniform distribution on A. Awkward shapes of region can be accommodated by simulating the process on a larger region of a more convenient shape, such as a rectangle or disc, and retaining only those events which lie within A. Note, in this context, that Hsuan (1979) gives an algorithm for the direct generation of events uniformly distributed on an arbitrary polygon.

If $N(A)$ is required to be randomly varying, this same method can of course be preceded by the simulation of $N(A)$ from the appropriate Poisson distribution. In some implementations, the direct simulation of $N(A)$ is a relatively time-consuming step. Lewis and Shedler (1979) propose an alternative method which can be used when A is a rectangle, say $A = (0, a) \times (0, b)$. This is based on the observation that the x-coordinates of events in the infinite strip $0 \leq y \leq b$ form a *one-dimensional* Poisson process with intensity λb, from which it follows that the differences between successive ordered x-coordinates are independent realizations of an exponentially distributed random variable with distribution function

$$F(v) = 1 - e^{-\lambda b v} \; : \; v > 0$$

(see, for example, Cox and Lewis, 1966, Chapter 2). The corresponding y-coordinates are, again independently, uniformly distributed on $(0, b)$. Note that this method automatically generates the events (x_i, y_i) in order of increasing x-coordinates, and terminates when the latest x-coordinate exceeds a.

4.5 Independence and random labelling

To assess the spatial association between the two types of events in a bivariate process, we can consider at least two different benchmark hypotheses:

(i) *independence* – where the two types of event are generated by a pair of independent univariate processes;
(ii) *random labelling* – where the two types of event are generated by labelling the events of a univariate process in a series of mutually independent Bernoulli trials.

These two hypotheses generate distinctively different K_{12}-functions.

Firstly, for any two independent processes of type 1 and type 2 events,

$$K_{12}(t) = \pi t^2.$$

This follows from the fact that, if the two component processes are independent, then an event of type 1 has the same status, with respect to events of type 2, as an arbitrary point, hence the expected number of type 2 events within a disc of radius t centred on an arbitrary type 1 event is $\lambda_2 \pi t^2$, the expected number of type 2 events per unit area multiplied by the area of the disc. It follows that $K_{12}(t) = \pi t^2$ as claimed.

Secondly, for any randomly labelled process of type 1 and type 2 events,

$$K_{11}(t) = K_{22}(t) = K_{12}(t) = K(t), \qquad (4.12)$$

where $K(s)$ is the K-function for the unlabelled univariate process. To see this, let $K(t)$ be the K-function of the unlabelled, univariate process consisting of all events, irrespective of type. Then, under random labelling the univariate processes of type 1 and type 2 events are each random thinnings of the unlabelled process, and we have already seen in Section 4.2.1 that the K-function is invariant under random thinning, hence $K_{11}(t) = K_{22}(t) = K(t)$. Essentially the same argument shows that $K_{12}(t) = K(t)$.

Note that independence and random labelling are equivalent if and only if the component processes of type 1 and type 2 events are both Poisson processes. This makes it important to decide which, if either, is the natural benchmark of 'no association' in a particular application.

4.6 Estimation of second-order properties

4.6.1 Univariate processes

For the reason given in Section 4.2, we shall focus on estimating the K-function. Given an estimate $\hat{K}(t)$, we can always use (4.3) to convert it to an estimate of $\lambda_2(t)$. Choose a bandwidth $h > 0$, make the approximation $\hat{K}'(t) \approx \{\hat{K}(t+h) - \hat{K}(t)\}/h$ and deduce the estimate

$$\hat{\lambda}_2(t) = \hat{\lambda}^2 (2\pi t)^{-1} \hat{K}'(t).$$

This produces a histogram-like estimate of $\lambda_2(t)$ at intervals of h in t. Stoyan and Stoyan (1994) discuss a kernel smoothing version, subsequently used by a number of authors including Møller et al. (1998).

In Section 4.2 we defined the function $K(t)$ by

$$\lambda K(t) = \mathrm{E}[N_0(t)],$$

the expected number of further events within distance t of an arbitrary event, where the intensity λ is the mean number of events per unit area. An obvious estimator for λ is the observed number of events per unit area, $\hat{\lambda} = n/|A|$.

Similarly, because $E(t) = \mathrm{E}[N_0(t)]$ is the expected number of further events within distance t of an arbitrary event, we can construct an estimator for $E(t)$ as follows. Let $u_{ij} = ||x_i - x_j||$. Define

$$\tilde{E}(t) = n^{-1} \sum_{i=1}^{n} \sum_{j \neq i} I(u_{ij} \leq t), \qquad (4.13)$$

where $I(\cdot)$ denotes the indicator function.

The form of the estimator $\tilde{E}(t)$ in (4.13) suggests, correctly, that the K-function is closely connected to the distribution of inter-event distances, whose use in exploratory analysis we discussed in Section 2.2. However, $\tilde{E}(t)$ is negatively biased for $E(t)$ because of edge effects. For a reference event within distance t of the boundary of A, the observed count of other events within distance t necessarily excludes any events

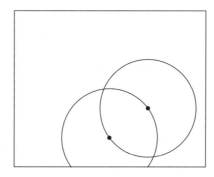

Figure 4.1. Construction of the edge-correction weights in Ripley's (1976) estimator for $K(t)$.

which may have occurred within distance t but outside A. Several methods have been proposed to correct for this source of bias; see, for example, Stein (1991) or Baddeley (1999). The following method, which we shall use in all of our examples, is due to Ripley (1976).

Let $w(x, u)$ be the proportion of the circumference of the circle with centre x and radius u which lies within A. Write w_{ij} for $w(x_i, u_{ij})$. Then, for any stationary isotropic process, w_{ij} is the conditional probability that an event is observed, given only that it is a distance u_{ij} away from the ith event x_i. See Figure 4.1, and note that in general $w_{ij} \neq w_{ji}$. Thus, an unbiased estimator for $E(t)$ is

$$\hat{E}(t) = n^{-1} \sum_{i=1}^{n} \sum_{j \neq i} w_{ij}^{-1} I_t(u_{ij}).$$

Finally, replacing the unknown intensity λ by $(n-1)/|A|$, we obtain Ripley's (1976) estimator for $K(t)$,

$$\hat{K}(t) = \{n(n-1)\}^{-1} |A| \sum_{i=1}^{n} \sum_{j \neq i} w_{ij}^{-1} I_t(u_{ij}). \tag{4.14}$$

In fact, Ripley used n^{-2} rather than $\{n(n-1)\}^{-1}$ in the expression for $\hat{K}(t)$; we prefer the given form for technical reasons, although the distinction is clearly unimportant when n is large.

Ripley's estimator is approximately unbiased for sufficiently small t, the restriction on t being necessary because the weights w_{ij} can become unbounded as t increases. In practice this is not a serious problem. For example, when A is the unit square the theoretical upper limit of t is $\frac{1}{2}\sqrt{2} \approx 0.7$ but $\hat{K}(t)$ will seldom be required for such large values of t, partly because the sampling fluctuations in $\hat{K}(t)$ increase with t but also because it is not realistic to attempt to model effects which operate on the same physical scale as the dimensions of A.

The Splancs software incorporates an algorithm, written by Barry Rowlingson, for computing $w(x, u)$ when A is an arbitrary polygon. Explicit formulae for $w(x, u)$ can also be written down for simple shapes of region A, for example rectangular or circular, and these may be useful if computational efficiency is paramount. Suppose, firstly, that A is the rectangle $(0, a) \times (0, b)$. Write $x = (x_1, x_2)$ and let $d_1 = \min(x_1, a - x_1)$, $d_2 = \min(x_2, b - x_2)$; thus d_1 and d_2 are the distances from the point x to the nearest vertical and horizontal edges of A. To calculate $w(x, u)$ we need to distinguish two cases:

1. if $u^2 \leq d_1^2 + d_2^2$, then

$$w(x, u) = 1 - \pi^{-1}[\cos^{-1}\{\min(d_1, u)/u\} + \cos^{-1}\{\min(d_2, u)/u\}]; \quad (4.15)$$

2. if $u^2 > d_1^2 + d_2^2$, then

$$w(x, u) = 0.75 - (2\pi)^{-1}\{\cos^{-1}(d_1/u) + \cos^{-1}(d_2/u)\}. \quad (4.16)$$

Note that (4.15) correctly gives $w(x, u) = 1$ when $u \leq \min(d_1, d_2)$. The above formulae apply to values of u in the range $0 \leq u \leq 0.5\min(a, b)$ which, as noted above, should be sufficient for practical purposes.

Now suppose that A is the disc with centre the origin and radius a. Let $r = \sqrt{(x_1^2 + x_2^2)}$ be the distance from x to the centre of the disc. Then, again distinguishing two cases, we have the following:

1. if $u \leq a - r$, then $w(x, u) = 1$;
2. if $u > a - r$, then $w(x, u) = 1 - \pi^{-1}\cos^{-1}\{(a^2 - r^2 - u^2)/(2ru)\}$.

These formulae apply to values of u between 0 and a.

The sampling distribution of $\hat{K}(t)$ is analytically intractable, except in the case of a homogeneous Poisson process. Given any specific model and region A, the sampling distribution can be estimated by direct simulation. However, the theoretical expression for the variance of $\hat{K}(t)$ in a homogeneous Poisson process provides a useful benchmark in initial inspection of a plot of $\hat{K}(t)$. In what follows, we treat n, the number of events in A, as fixed.

For a homogeneous Poisson process, Ripley (1988) gives an asymptotic approximation to the sampling variance of $\hat{K}(t)$. Lotwick and Silverman (1982) give exact formulae whose evaluation in general requires extensive numerical integration, although they give explicit formulae for rectangular A. Chetwynd and Diggle (1998) give a different approximation, based on a thinning argument, which is easily computed for arbitrarily shaped A.

Ripley's asymptotic approximation, modified to take account of our non-standard choice of denominator in (4.14), is

$$v_R(t) = 2\{|A|/(n-1)\}^2\{\pi t^2/|A| + 0.96Pt^3/|A|^2 \\ + 0.13(n/|A|)Pt^5/|A|^2\}, \quad (4.17)$$

where P denotes the perimeter of A. The approximation is accurate for relatively small values of t (see below).

Lotwick and Silverman's result, similarly modified and assuming rectangular A, is that the variance of $\hat{K}(t)$ is

$$v_{LS}(t) = \{n(n-1)\}^{-1}\{2b(t) - a_1(t) + (n-2)a_2(t)\}, \quad (4.18)$$

where, for rectangular A with perimeter length P,

$$b(t) = \pi t^2 |A|^{-1}(1 - \pi t^2/|A|) + |A|^{-2}(1.0716Pt^2 + 2.2375t^4),$$

$$a_1(t) = |A|^{-2}(0.21Pt^3 + 1.3t^4)$$

and

$$a_2(t) = |A|^{-3}(0.24Pt^5 + 2.62t^6).$$

These expressions are valid for t less than or equal to the shorter side-length of A.

Chetwynd and Diggle's approximation involves summations of functions of the edge-correction weights w_{ij} as follows. For any fixed t, define $\phi_{ij} = 0.5(w_{ij} + w_{ji})I(||x_i - x_j|| \leq t)$. Further define

$$W_n = \sum_{i=1}^{n} \sum_{j \neq i} \phi_{ij},$$

$$X_n = \sum_{i=1}^{n} \sum_{j \neq i} \phi_{ij}^2$$

and

$$Z_n = \sum_{i=1}^{n} \left(\sum_{j \neq i} \phi_{ij} \right)^2.$$

Write $n^{(k)} = n(n-1) \cdots (n-k+1)$ and define $m_2(t) = X_n/n^{(2)}$, $m_3(t) = (Z_n - X_n)/n^{(3)}$ and $m_4(t) = (W_n^2 - 4Z_n + 2X_n)/n^{(4)}$. Then the estimated variance of $\hat{K}(t)$ is

$$v_{CD}(t) = (2|A|^2/n^{(2)})\{(3 - 2n)m_4(t) + 2(n - 2)m_3(t) + m_2(t)\}. \qquad (4.19)$$

Chetwynd and Diggle in fact give an explicit formula for $\text{Cov}\{\hat{K}(t), \hat{K}(s)\}$, of which (4.19) is a special case.

It is also useful to be able to assess the precision of an estimate of $K(t)$ without assuming a specific model. A simple way to do this is to subdivide A into equal sub-areas, estimate $K(t)$ separately within each sub-area and use the empirical variance over the separate estimates. Thus, if for each t we let k_i denote the estimate of $K(t)$ from the ith of m sub-areas, then our overall estimate is

$$\tilde{K}(t) = m^{-1} \sum_{i=1}^{m} k_i \qquad (4.20)$$

with approximate variance

$$\text{Var}\{\tilde{K}(t)\} \approx \{(m(m-1)\}^{-1} \sum_{i=1}^{m} \{k_i - \tilde{K}(t)\}^2. \qquad (4.21)$$

Note that the approximation in (4.21) arises for two reasons. Firstly, an element of approximation is inherent in using the sample variance of the k_i as an estimate of their true variance; secondly, dividing the sample variance of the k_i by m makes the implicit assumption that disjoint sub-regions give independent estimates k_i, which is correct for the homogeneous Poisson process, but not more generally. Furthermore, $\tilde{K}(t)$ can be expected to be less efficient than $\hat{K}(t)$ because it does not use information from pairs of events in different sub-regions; this may be an important consideration unless n, the number of events, is very large. All of these considerations suggest that the estimator $\tilde{K}(t)$ and its associated approximate variance should be used only for relatively small values of t, or when the artificial subdivision of A is replaced by genuine replication. We postpone further discussion of replicated patterns until Chapter 8.

We now illustrate the performance of the different estimators for $\mathrm{Var}\{\hat{K}(s)\}$. We consider first the homogeneous Poisson process. Figure 4.2 shows the ratio of Ripley's asymptotic approximation (4.17) and the Lotwick–Silverman formula (4.18), for $n = 100$, 200 and 400, and A the unit square. For small t, the approximation is excellent when $n = 100$ and, as would be expected, improves as n increases. At larger values of t, it is less reliable and does not necessarily improve as n increases. For a comparison between the Lotwick–Silverman formula and the Chetwynd–Diggle method, we need to simulate replicate patterns because the latter is a data-based estimate rather than a numerical approximation. Figure 4.3 is comparable to Figure 4.2 except that the comparison is now between the Chetwynd–Diggle estimated variance, averaged over replicate simulations, and the Lotwick–Silverman formula. The results point to a small negative bias in the Chetwynd–Diggle estimator at large distances.

In a second experiment, we again simulated homogeneous Poisson processes but now compared the two estimators $\hat{K}(t)$ and $\tilde{K}(t)$, the latter using a subdivision of the unit square into a 4×4 grid of smaller squares. The results summarized below are based on 1000 replicates of processes with each of $n = 100$, 200 and 400 events on the unit square, and for distances $t \leq 0.25$.

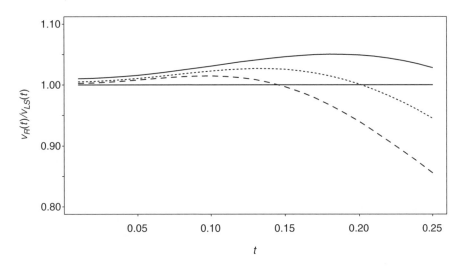

Figure 4.2. Comparison between Ripley's asymptotic approximation and the Lotwick–Silverman formula for the sampling variance of $\hat{K}(t)$: $n = 100$ (solid curve); $n = 200$ (dashed curve); $n = 400$ (dotted curve). The horizontal line at height 1 corresponds to equality of the two formulae.

54   Statistical analysis of spatial point patterns

Recall that for the homogeneous Poisson process, the implicit assumption in (4.21) that disjoint sub-regions give independent estimates of $K(t)$ is correct, and the simulations confirmed this. Perhaps more interestingly, Figure 4.4 shows the ratio of the estimated variance of $\tilde{K}(t)$ and the Lotwick–Silverman formula $v_{LS}(t)$ for the variance of $\hat{K}(t)$. This confirms the inherent inefficiency of $\tilde{K}(t)$ relative to $\hat{K}(t)$, especially for small n and/or large t.

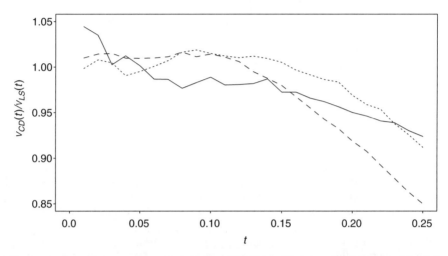

Figure 4.3. Comparison between Chetwynd and Diggle's estimator and the Lotwick–Silverman formula for the sampling variance of $\hat{K}(t)$: $n = 100$ (solid curve); $n = 200$ (dashed curve); $n = 400$ (dotted curve).

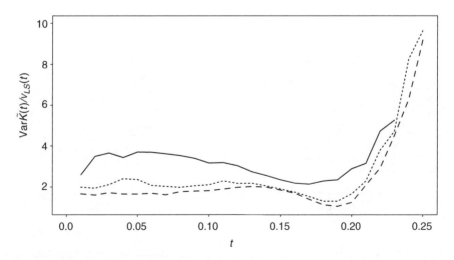

Figure 4.4. Comparison between the variances of $\tilde{K}(t)$ and of $\hat{K}(t)$: $n = 100$ (solid curve); $n = 200$ (dotted curve); $n = 400$ (dashed curve).

Finally, we simulated two non-Poisson processes, one generating aggregated patterns similar to Figure 1.2, the other regular patterns with a minimum permissible distance between events, similar to Figure 1.3. The results confirm that, as expected, formulae based on a Poisson assumption tend to underestimate or overestimate the variance of $\hat{K}(t)$ according to whether the underlying process is aggregated or regular, respectively. Specifically, in the aggregated case the estimated variances were between two and 12 times larger than the Poisson-based Lotwick–Silverman formulae, and in the regular case between three and seven times smaller over the range $t \leq 0.25$ (excluding small distances for which $\hat{K}(t)$ is identically zero because of the minimum permissible inter-event distance). However, the approximation (4.21) continued to give reasonable estimates for the variance of the less efficient estimator $\tilde{K}(t)$.

Our overall conclusions from these comparisons are the following. For the initial exploration of second-order structure of patterns which are close to completely random, it is useful to supplement a graphical display of $\hat{K}(t)$ with error bounds based on the Lotwick–Silverman formula for rectangular regions, or using the Chetwynd–Diggle formula for regions with an irregular boundary, such as arise typically in epidemiological applications. For patterns markedly different from completely random, Poisson-based approximations are unreliable. When a parametric model has been formulated, standard errors can be estimated from repeated simulation of the declared model. In the absence of a parametric model, the less efficient estimator $\tilde{K}(t)$ can be used if a reliable indication of precision is required.

4.6.2 Inhomogeneous processes

If we assume that the process is reweighted stationary and, unrealistically, that the first-order intensity $\lambda(x)$ is known, we can estimate $K_I(t)$ by an easy modification of (4.17). The modification consists of rescaling the inter-event distances by the product of the first-order intensities at the corresponding two locations, leading to the estimator

$$\hat{K}_I(t;\lambda) = |A|^{-1} \sum_{i=1}^{n} \sum_{j \neq i} w_{ij}^{-1} I_t(u_{ij})/\{\lambda(x_i)\lambda(x_j)\}. \qquad (4.22)$$

This was proposed by Baddeley et al. (2000), who went on to discuss the consequences of using an estimated first-order intensity $\hat{\lambda}(x)$ in place of the true $\lambda(x)$. Unsurprisingly, this introduces difficulties in practice, because of the difficulty of distinguishing empirically between non-constancy of $\lambda(x)$ and dependence between the events of the process. This relates to the equivalence of certain classes of Cox process and Poisson cluster process, to be discussed in Chapter 5. As a consequence, it is difficult in practice simultaneously to estimate non-parametrically both first-order and second-order properties of a reweighted stationary process. One situation in which it is easier to disentangle first-order and second-order properties is in the analysis of case–control data in epidemiology. We discuss this in Section 9.7.

4.6.3 Multivariate processes

To estimate $K_{12}(s)$ for a bivariate pattern we use the same basic idea as in estimating $K(s)$, but measure distances between pairs of events of different types. Thus, if u_{ij} is the distance between the ith event of type 1 and the jth event of type 2, w_{ij} is as before, and the numbers of type 1 and type 2 events are n_1 and n_2 respectively, we can construct two estimates of $\hat{K}_{12}(s)$ as follows:

(i) $\hat{\lambda}_2 \tilde{K}_{12}(s) = n_1^{-1} \sum_{i=1}^{n_1} \sum_{j=1}^{n_2} w_{ij} I(u_{ij} \leq s),$

(ii) $\hat{\lambda}_1 \tilde{K}_{21}(s) = n_2^{-1} \sum_{j=1}^{n_2} \sum_{i=1}^{n_1} w_{ji} I(u_{ij} \leq s).$

We then combine the two estimates as a weighted average, to give

$$\hat{K}_{12}(s) = (n_1 n_2)^{-1} |A| \left\{ n_1 \sum_{i=1}^{n_1} \sum_{j=1}^{n_2} w_{ij} I(u_{ij} \leq s) \right.$$
$$\left. + n_2 \sum_{j=1}^{n_2} \sum_{i=1}^{n_1} w_{ji} I(u_{ij} \leq s) \right\} \Big/ (n_1 + n_2)$$
$$= (n_1 n_2)^{-1} |A| \sum_{i=1}^{n_1} \sum_{j=1}^{n_2} w^*_{ij} I(u_{ij} \leq s), \qquad (4.23)$$

where

$$w^*_{ij} = (n_1 w_{ij} + n_2 w_{ji})/(n_1 + n_2).$$

The variance formulae in Lotwick and Silverman (1982) include the bivariate case. In addition to the functions $v(t)$, $a_1(t)$ and $a_2(t)$ defined above, let $c = n_2/(n_1 + n_2)$. Then, when the component processes are independent homogeneous Poisson processes,

$$\text{Var}\{\hat{K}_{12}(t)\} = (n_1 n_2)^{-1} |A|^2 [v(t) - 2c(1-c)a_1(t)$$
$$+ \{(n_1 - 1)c^2 + (n_2 - 1)(1 - c)^2\} a_2(t)]. \qquad (4.24)$$

4.6.4 Examples

Figure 4.5 shows the estimate $\hat{D}(t) = \hat{K}(t) - \pi t^2$ for the Japanese black pine sapling data of Figure 1.1, together with plus and minus two standard deviation limits calculated from the Lotwick–Silverman formula under the assumption that the data are generated by a homogeneous Poisson process. Note that $\hat{D}(t)$ lies within these limits throughout the plotted range, suggesting compatibility with the Poisson assumption as in earlier analyses of these data.

Note also that the standard deviation under the Poisson assumption is roughly linear in t. This is an indirect consequence of the Poisson quadrat count distribution, since $\hat{K}(t)$ is essentially an average of counts in circles of radius t, hence its mean and variance are both approximately proportional to t^2. For this reason, some authors recommend plotting $\sqrt{\hat{K}(t)}$ against t to stabilize the sampling variance, and incidentally to linearize the plot under the Poisson assumption. We prefer to plot $\hat{D}(t)$ because of its direct physical interpretation in terms of counting numbers of events in circular regions; also,

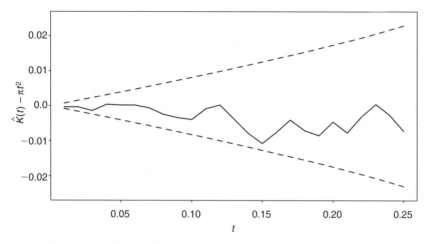

Figure 4.5. The estimate $\hat{K}(t) - \pi t^2$ for the Japanese black pine data: data (solid curve); plus and minus two standard errors under CSR (dashed curves).

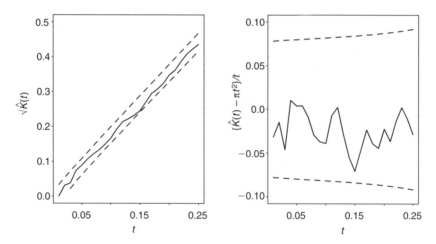

Figure 4.6. Transformed estimates of $\hat{K}(t)$ for the Japanese black pine data: data (solid curve); plus and minus two standard errors under CSR (dashed curves). $\sqrt{\hat{K}(t)}$ is shown on the left, $\{\hat{K}(t) - \pi t^2\}/t$ on the right.

as we shall show in later chapters, plots of $D(t)$ can be used for preliminary estimation of parameters for some widely used models. If a variance-stable plot is required, either the square-root scale can be used, or a standardized difference, $\hat{D}(t)/t$, although the latter would become numerically unstable if extrapolated to $t = 0$. The two panels of Figure 4.6 show these two plots for the Japanese black pine data. In each case, the error limits are obtained by the appropriate transformation of the plus and minus two standard error limits for $\hat{K}(t)$ calculated by the Lotwick–Silverman formula.

The two panels of Figure 4.7 show $\hat{D}(t)$ with plus and minus two standard error limits under complete spatial randomness, for the redwood data of Figure 1.2, and for

58 Statistical analysis of spatial point patterns

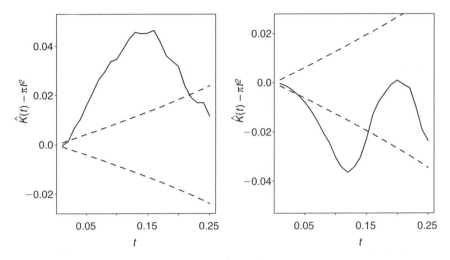

Figure 4.7. The estimate $\hat{D}(t) = \hat{K}(t) - \pi t^2$ for the redwood data (left) and for the cell data (right): data (solid curve); plus and minus two standard errors under CSR (dashed curves).

the cell data of Figure 1.3. In contrast to Figure 4.5, it is clear in both cases that the data are incompatible with complete spatial randomness, but for opposite reasons. As is now very familiar, the redwood data display strong spatial aggregation, and the cell data strong spatial regularity. Note that the damped oscillatory behaviour of $\hat{D}(t)$ for the cell data is typical of regular patterns.

4.7 Displaced amacrine cells in the retina of a rabbit

The displaced amacrine cell data, shown in Figure 1.4, illustrate how estimated K-functions can be used in a specific context without explicit parametric modelling. The analysis presented here is adapted from Diggle (1985a).

The primary scientific interest in these data is to distinguish between two developmental hypotheses (Hughes, 1981). Recall that the two types of cell are those which respond to a light being switched *on* or *off*, respectively. The *separate layer* hypothesis is that the on and off cells are initially formed in two separate layers which later fuse to form the mature retina, whilst the *single layer* hypothesis is that the two types of cell are initially undifferentiated in a single layer and acquire their separate functions at a later stage.

Figure 4.8 shows estimates of $K_{ij}(t)$ for each of $(i, j) = (1, 1), (1, 2)$ and $(2, 2)$, where types 1 and 2 refer to on and off cells, respectively, and of $K(t)$ for the superposition of both types of cell. Note, firstly, that the estimate of $K_{12}(t) - \pi t^2$ is close to zero throughout the plotted range. We could use the Lotwick–Silverman formula to compute the sampling variance of $K_{12}(t)$ under the assumption that the two types of cell form independent Poisson processes, but this is likely to overestimate the variance because, as shown by the estimates of $K_{11}(t)$ and $K_{22}(t)$, the component patterns are markedly more regular than the Poisson process. However, we can test the independence hypothesis using a procedure also suggested by Lotwick and Silverman

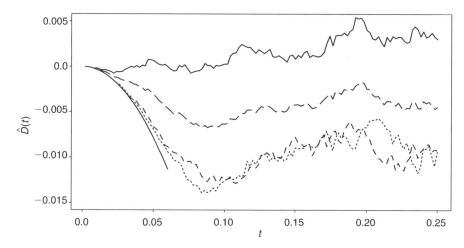

Figure 4.8. Second-order properties of displaced amacrine cells. Functions plotted are $\hat{D}(t) = \hat{K}(t) - \pi t^2$ as follows: on cells (shorter-dashed curve); off cells (dotted curve); all cells (longer-dashed curve); bivariate (solid curve). The parabola $-\pi t^2$ is also shown as a solid line.

(1982). If we wrap the rectangular observation window A onto a torus, independence of the component processes would imply that the sampling distribution of $\hat{K}_{12}(t)$ is invariant to a random toroidal shift of either pattern. This in turn implies that we can conduct a Monte Carlo test of independence by comparing the value of a suitable test statistic for the observed data with values generated under a sequence of independent random toroidal shifts. Using the test statistic

$$u = \sum_{k=1}^{125} t_k^{-2} \{\hat{K}_{12}(t_k) - \pi t_k^2\}^2,$$

where $t_k = 0.002, 0.004, \ldots, 0.250$, we implemented a Monte Carlo test by recalculating u after each of 99 independent random toroidal shifts, and obtained a p-value of 0.12. Thus, at least with regard to their second-order properties, the evidence against the hypothesis of independent components is weak. This is supportive of the separate layer hypothesis. However, the evidence is not yet conclusive since the result that $K_{12}(t) = \pi t^2$ is necessary, but not sufficient, for independence.

We now examine $\hat{K}_{11}(t)$ and $\hat{K}_{22}(t)$, and note that they are very similar to each other, but markedly different from $\hat{K}(t)$ for the superposition. This suggests that if the observed pattern is the result of a labelling of an initially undifferentiated set of cells, then the labelling cannot be random. We could formally test the hypothesis of random labelling, but this seems unnecessary in view of the very clear difference between $\hat{K}(t)$ for the superposition and the two very similar estimates $\hat{K}_{11}(t)$ and $\hat{K}_{22}(t)$.

The argument so far leaves open the possibility that the observed pattern is the result of a non-random labelling process. However, note that both $\hat{K}_{11}(t)$ and $\hat{K}_{22}(t)$ are zero for $t < 0.025$ approximately, whereas $\hat{K}(t)$ for the superposition is non-zero at much smaller values of t. For this to arise from a labelling process, the following would have

60 *Statistical analysis of spatial point patterns*

to be true: in the undifferentiated process, close pairs of cells are allowed but mutually close triples are forbidden; and in the labelling process, the two members of a close pair must always be oppositely labelled. This seems implausible, and the analysis therefore points strongly towards the separate layer hypothesis being the correct explanation.

4.8 Estimation of nearest neighbour distributions

We now consider estimation of the two nearest neighbour distribution functions introduced in Sections 2.3 and 2.4. These are $F(x)$, the probability that the distance from an arbitrary point to the nearest event is less than or equal to x; and $G(x)$, the probability that the distance from an arbitrary event to the nearest other event is less than or equal to x.

In either case, the simplest estimator is the empirical distribution function of observed nearest neighbour distances, as used in Sections 2.3 and 2.4. These estimators are biased because of edge effects. The bias does not affect the validity of a Monte Carlo test of CSR, or indeed of any other specified model, but would be problematic if we were directly concerned with estimation.

One approach to edge correction is the following, due to Ripley (1977). Consider first an estimator for $G(y)$. Let $(y_i, d_i) : i = 1, \ldots, n$ denote the distances from each event to the nearest other event in A and to the nearest point on the boundary of A, respectively, and define the estimator $\tilde{G}(y)$ to be the proportion of nearest neighbour distances $y_i \leq y$ amongst those events at least a distance y from the boundary of A; thus

$$\tilde{G}(y) = \#(y_i \leq y, d_i > y)/\#(d_i > y).$$

To estimate $F(x)$, similarly let $(x_i, e_i) : i = 1, \ldots, m$ denote the distances from each of m sample points to the nearest event in A and to the nearest point on the boundary of A, and define

$$\tilde{F}(x) = \#(x_i \leq x, e_i > x)/\#(e_i > x).$$

As in Section 2.4, for estimation of $F(x)$ we would suggest locating the m sample points in a regular grid. Alternatively, we could avoid altogether the need for a grid of sample points by computing directly the areal proportion of the study region for which the distance to the nearest event is less than or equal to x (Lotwick, 1981).

A technically simpler procedure for dealing with edge effects would be to use the buffer-zone method, taking measurements only from points or events sufficiently far from the boundary of A, so that edge effects do not arise for the range of distances of interest. As noted in Section 1.3, the obvious disadvantage of this procedure is that it effectively throws away a non-trivial proportion of the data.

Recall also from Section 2.7 that Van Lieshout and Baddeley's J-function, defined by $J(x) = \{1 - G(x)\}/\{1 - F(x)\}$, can be estimated reliably without any correction for edge effects.

The sampling distributions of estimators for $F(\cdot)$ and $G(\cdot)$ appear to be intractable, although for large data-sets the device of splitting the observation region A into subregions to form pseudo-replicates is available, whilst simulation can be used to assess the fit of a parametric model.

4.8.1 Examples

Figure 4.9 compares the empirical distribution functions, $\hat{G}(\cdot)$ and $\hat{F}(\cdot)$, with the edge-corrected estimators $\tilde{G}(\cdot)$ and $\tilde{F}(\cdot)$ for the Japanese black pine sapling data of Figure 1.1. Notice that the two estimates in each case are very similar, but that the edge-corrected estimators are not necessarily monotone.

Figures 4.10 and 4.11 are the corresponding plots for the redwood seedling data of Figure 1.2 and for the cell data of Figure 1.3. For comparability, all six plots in

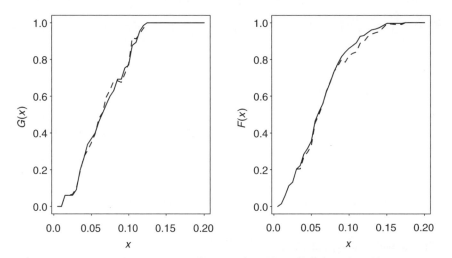

Figure 4.9. Estimates of F(x) (right) and G(x) (left) for the Japanese black pine data: the solid curve is $\hat{G}(\cdot)$, $\hat{F}(\cdot)$; the dashed one is $\tilde{G}(\cdot)$, $\tilde{F}(\cdot)$.

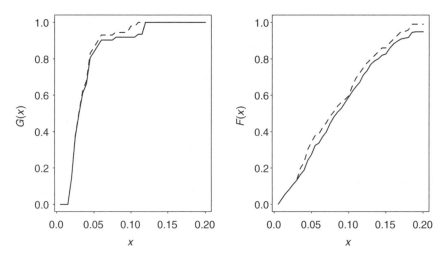

Figure 4.10. Estimates of F(x) (right) and G(x) (left) for the redwood data: the solid curve is $\hat{G}(\cdot)$, $\hat{F}(\cdot)$; the dashed one is $\tilde{G}(\cdot)$, $\tilde{F}(\cdot)$.

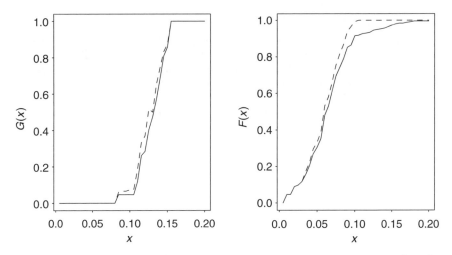

Figure 4.11. Estimates of $F(x)$ (right) and $G(x)$ (left) for the cell data: the solid curve is $\hat{G}(\cdot)$, $\hat{F}(\cdot)$; the dashed one is $\tilde{G}(\cdot)$, $\tilde{F}(\cdot)$.

Figures 4.9, 4.10 and 4.11 evaluate the estimates over the same set of distances. The qualitative differences amongst these three data-sets are again clear.

4.9 Concluding remarks

The K-function, and the two nearest neighbour distribution functions $F(\cdot)$ and $G(\cdot)$, provide complementary tools for the description of spatial point processes.

The K-function is the most amenable of the three to theoretical analysis. We shall see in later chapters that its algebraic form can be derived for a number of useful models. Its physical interpretation as a scaled expectation is also a useful property. The sampling distribution of its estimator $\hat{K}(t)$ is reasonably well understood in the case of a homogeneous Poisson process, but otherwise must be assessed by splitting the observation region into sub-regions, or by simulation.

All three functions are useful for an exploratory assessment of departure from CSR. More generally, we shall see in later chapters that the estimated K-function is a useful and versatile tool. In the author's opinion, the principal use of estimates of $F(\cdot)$ and $G(\cdot)$ is to provide goodness-of-fit measures which are complementary to the second-order description provided by the K-function. In this respect, it is worth noting that the function $J(x) = \{1 - G(x)\}/\{1 - F(x)\}$ can sometimes be calculated explicitly when its separate components $F(x)$ and $G(x)$ are intractable.

5
Models

5.1 Introduction

The basic building block for point process modelling is the Poisson process. As discussed in Chapter 4, the homogeneous Poisson process provides a benchmark of complete spatial randomness (CSR) against which various kinds of pattern can be assessed. The essence of CSR is that events are located independently of each other. When the occurrence of an event at a particular location makes it more likely that other events will be located nearby, the resulting patterns display a kind of pattern which might loosely be described as *aggregated*. In contrast, when each event is likely to be surrounded by empty space, the overall pattern will be of a more *regular* spatial distribution of events.

In the remainder of this chapter, we will describe some simple constructions for these and other, more complex types of spatial pattern.

5.2 Contagious distributions

Historically, the first extension of the Poisson process as a model for spatial point patterns was advanced by Neyman (1939), who was concerned with possible models for the spatial distribution of insect larvae. Neyman postulated a Poisson process of egg-masses from which larvae hatch and subsequently move to positions relative to the corresponding egg-mass according to a bivariate distribution with pdf $h(\cdot)$. The probability that a larva from an egg-mass at x will subsequently be found within a region A is

$$P(x; A) = \int_A h(y - z) dy.$$

Neyman then argued that without any knowledge of $h(\cdot)$ a model might reasonably be specified by a prescribed form for $P(x; A)$. However, Skellam (1958) subsequently pointed out that the implied integral equation for $h(\cdot)$ may not be soluble; note that the required solution is a pdf which must not depend on A.

Rather more simply, suppose that 'parent' events form a Poisson process with intensity ρ and that each parent independently produces a random number S of 'offspring', all of which occupy the *same* position as their parent. The number of parents, M say, in a given region A therefore follows a Poisson distribution with mean $\rho|A|$. The number of offspring in A, $N(A)$ say, is $S_1 + \cdots + S_M$, and if the probability generating function (pgf) of S is $\pi_s(z)$, then the pgf of $N(A)$ is

$$\pi(z; A) = \exp\left[-\rho|A|\{1 - \pi_s(z)\}\right]. \tag{5.1}$$

Equation (5.1) defines the class of *generalized* Poisson distributions (Feller, 1968, Chapter 12, but note the difference in terminology). In the present context, such distributions are usually called *contagious*, following Neyman (1939). Neyman's Type A distribution is obtained by setting $\pi_s(z) = \exp\{-\mu(1 - z)\}$ and therefore corresponds to a non-orderly process of randomly distributed *point clusters*. A variation due to Thomas (1949) is to include parents in the final pattern. This avoids 'clusters' of zero size and corresponds to $\pi_s(z) = z \exp\{-\mu(1 - z)\}$. Finally, if S has a logarithmic series distribution with $\pi_s(z) = 1 - \log\{1 + \beta(1 - z)\}/\log(1 + \beta)$, for some $\beta > 0$, then Y has a negative binomial distribution. The absence of any genuinely spatial clustering mechanism in the formulation of these contagious distributions should be noted. Furthermore, it is well known that the negative binomial distribution in particular can be derived also as a *compounded*, or mixed, Poisson distribution in which the parameter of a Poisson distribution is determined by random sampling from a gamma distribution.

Contagious distributions have long been fitted to quadrat count data, with apparent success. Evans (1953) gives a number of ecological examples, whilst Douglas (1979) contains a detailed description of the relevant statistical methodology. This approach provides at best an empirical description of *pattern*, and specific inferences about the underlying *process* should be avoided. In particular, it is far from clear that a negative binomial quadrat count distribution can be compatible with any spatial point process other than a point cluster process of the type defined by (5.1) or a non-ergodic process in which each complete realization is a Poisson process, but whose intensity λ varies between realizations according to a gamma distribution; see, for example, the discussion of Matérn (1971).

The existence question was pursued by Diggle and Milne (1983a), who tried and failed to find a construction for which the resulting point process was stationary, ergodic, orderly and with negative binomial quadrat count distributions. They conjectured that no such process exists, and this was subsequently confirmed in unpublished work by Bob Griffiths (Department of Statistics, University of Oxford).

5.3 Poisson cluster processes

Poisson cluster processes, introduced by Neyman and Scott (1958), incorporate an explicit form of spatial clustering, and therefore provide a more satisfactory basis for modelling aggregated spatial point patterns. Their definition incorporates the following three postulates:

PCP1 Parent events form a Poisson process with intensity ρ.
PCP2 Each parent produces a random number S of offspring, realized independently and identically for each parent according to a probability distribution p_s : $s = 0, 1, \ldots$.
PCP3 The positions of the offspring relative to their parents are independently and identically distributed according to a bivariate pdf $h(\cdot)$.

Conventionally, and in the sequel unless explicitly stated otherwise, the final pattern consists of the offspring only. Some authors adopt a less restrictive definition involving the superposition of independent realizations of an arbitrary process, translated by the points of a Poisson parent process.

Poisson cluster processes as defined here are stationary, with intensity $\lambda = \rho\mu$ where $\mu = E[S]$. They are isotropic if PCP3 specifies a radially symmetric pdf $h(\cdot)$.

To express the second-order properties in terms of the three postulates PCP1 to PCP3, let

$$h_2(x) = \int h(x)h(x-y)dx$$

be the pdf of the vector difference between the positions of two offspring from the same parent, and $H_2(\cdot)$ the corresponding cumulative distribution function. If we now consider an arbitrary event within a cluster of size S, the expected number of other events from the same cluster within a distance t is $(S-1)H_2(t)$. The probability distribution of the size of the cluster to which an arbitrary event belongs is obtained by length-biased sampling from the cluster size distribution $p(s)$, hence $p^*(s) = sp(s)/\mu$: $s = 1, \ldots$. Averaging over the distribution $p^*(\cdot)$ then gives the expected number of related events within distance t of an arbitrary event as $E[S(S-1)]H_2(t)/\mu$.

Now consider the expected number of unrelated events, meaning events from different clusters, within distance t of an arbitrary event. PCP1 implies that all such events are located independently of the original event, hence their expected number is just $\lambda\pi t^2$.

Summing the contributions from related and unrelated events then gives

$$\lambda K(t) = \lambda\pi t^2 + E[S(S-1)]H_2(t)/\mu.$$

Finally, dividing by $\lambda = \rho\mu$, we obtain

$$K(t) = \pi t^2 + E[S(S-1)]H_2(t)/(\rho\mu^2). \qquad (5.2)$$

Differentiation of (5.2), in conjunction with (4.3), then gives

$$\lambda_2(t) = \lambda^2 + \rho E[S(S-1)]h_2(t). \qquad (5.3)$$

Note that the second term on the right-hand side of (5.2) is non-negative, and monotone non-decreasing, and that $K(t) - \pi t^2$ approaches a constant, $c = E[S(S-1)]/(\rho\mu^2)$, as $t \to \infty$. If S follows a Poisson distribution, $c = \rho^{-1}$. These results suggest a useful way of identifying whether a Poisson cluster process might be a reasonable model for an observed pattern, and if so a means of obtaining preliminary parameter estimates.

The variance of the quadrat count distribution for a Poisson cluster process is similarly obtained from (4.5) and (5.3) as

$$\text{Var}\{N(A)\} = \rho\mu|A| + \rho E[S(S-1)]\int_A\int_A h_2(x-y)dx\,dy.$$

General expressions for the nearest neighbour distributions of an isotropic Poisson cluster process are also available (Bartlett, 1975, Chapter 1). In the isotropic case, let $q(x, y)$ denote the probability that there are no offspring within a distance x of the origin, from a parent a distance y from the origin. Then the distribution function of the point-to-nearest-event distance is

$$F(x) = 1 - \exp\left(-2\pi\rho \int_0^\infty \{1 - q(x, y)\} y \, dy\right).$$

Because parents' locations are mutually independent, the distribution function of nearest neighbour distance follows immediately as

$$G(y) = 1 - \{1 - F(y)\} q^*(y),$$

where $q^*(y)$ denotes the probability that no offspring from the same parent as an arbitrary offspring, O say, lie within a distance y of O. In principle, the probabilities $q(x, y)$ and $q^*(y)$ are expressible in terms of the distributions specified in PCP2 and PCP3. Whilst the general expressions are not particularly illuminating, explicit results are obtainable in special cases; see, for example, Warren (1971) and Diggle (1975, 1978). Note also that $q^*(y)$ is an example of Van Lieshout and Baddeley's (1996) J-function.

In simulating Poisson cluster processes on a rectangular region, say $A = (0, a) \times (0, b)$, a useful device to avoid edge effects is to impose periodic boundary conditions. Parents in A are first generated as a partial realization of the appropriate Poisson process, as described in Section 4.4. Offspring are now attached to parents according to PCP2 and located according to PCP3, with the following exceptions:

1. Any generated x-coordinate of the form $ka + x$, for non-zero integer k and $0 < x < a$, is transformed to x.
2. Any generated y-coordinate of the form $kb + y$, for non-zero integer k and $0 < y < b$, is transformed to y.

In effect, the rectangle is converted to a torus by identifying opposite edges.

When PCP2 specifies a Poisson distribution for the number of offspring per parent, the process can, if required, be simulated conditional on the total number of events in A by randomly allocating the events amongst the parents. Conditioning on the number of parents in A is straightforward.

Figure 5.1 shows a realization of a process with 25 parents on the unit square and four offspring per parent. The position of each offspring relative to its parent follows a radially symmetric Gaussian distribution with pdf

$$h(x_1, x_2) = (2\pi\sigma^2)^{-1} \exp\{-(x_1^2 + x_2^2)/2\sigma^2\}$$

and $\sigma = 0.025$. Notice that because formally distinct clusters coalesce it is difficult to identify the 25 sets of four offspring with any confidence. Figure 5.2 shows a parallel realization in which the 100 offspring are randomly allocated amongst the 25 parents. Both patterns have used the same locations for parents, but the additional random element in Figure 5.2 makes it still more difficult to identify the underlying process by visual inspection.

Poisson cluster processes can be extended to 'multi-generation' processes in which the offspring become the parents of the next generation, and so on. This type of construction tends to be mathematically intractable, but it is intuitively appealing and we shall discuss it further in Section 5.5.

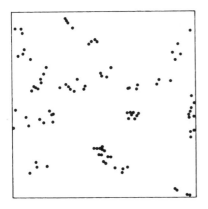 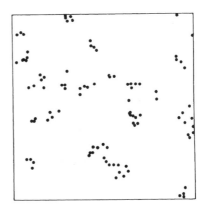

Figure 5.1. A realization of a Poisson cluster process with 25 parents on the unit square, 4 offspring per parent and radially symmetric Gaussian dispersion of offspring, with parameter $\sigma = 0.025$.

Figure 5.2. A realization of a Poisson cluster process with 100 offspring randomly allocated amongst 25 parents on the unit square and radially symmetric Gaussian dispersion of offspring, with parameter $\sigma = 0.025$.

5.4 Inhomogeneous Poisson processes

A class of *non-stationary* point processes is obtained if the constant intensity λ of the Poisson process is replaced by a spatially varying intensity function, $\lambda(x)$. This defines the class of inhomogeneous Poisson processes with the following properties:

IPP1 $N(A)$ has a Poisson distribution with mean $\int_A \lambda(x)dx$.
IPP2 Given $N(A) = n$, the n events in A form an independent random sample from the distribution on A with pdf proportional to $\lambda(x)$.

Figure 5.3 shows a partial realization of an inhomogeneous Poisson process with A the unit square, $N(A) = 100$ and $\lambda(x_1, x_2) = \exp(-2x_1 - x_2)$. The intensity gradient in the x_1-direction is immediately apparent, the gentler gradient in the x_2-direction less so.

The inhomogeneous Poisson process provides a possible framework for the introduction of covariates into the analysis of spatial point patterns via an intensity function $\lambda(x) = \lambda\{z_1(x), z_2(x), \ldots, z_p(x)\}$. For example, suppose that the locations of trees of a particular species is thought to follow a Poisson process with intensity determined by height above sea-level; then a possible model might be $\lambda(x) = \exp\{\alpha + \beta z(x)\}$, where $z(x)$ denotes height above sea-level at the location x. Cox (1972) refers to this as a 'modulated Poisson process'.

Another example, which we will consider in more detail in Chapter 9, is a model for the point process of cases of a respiratory disease in the vicinity of a point source of environmental pollution. In this example, we might assume that case locations form an inhomogeneous Poisson process with intensity $\lambda(x)$ given by

$$\lambda(x) = \lambda_0(x) f\{||x - x_0||, \theta\},$$

68 Statistical analysis of spatial point patterns

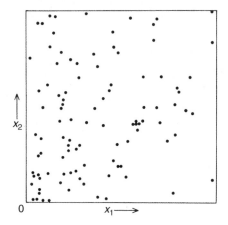

Figure 5.3. A realization of an inhomogeneous Poisson process with 100 events on the unit square and $\lambda(x) = \exp(-2x_1 - x_2)$.

where $\lambda_0(x)$ corresponds to spatial variation in population density, x_0 is the location of the point source, and $f(u, \theta)$ describes how the impact of the source varies with distance, u.

Provided that $\lambda(x)$ is bounded away from zero, inhomogeneous Poisson processes are reweighted second-order stationary in the sense of Baddeley *et al.* (2000), with reweighted second-order intensity $\rho(t) = 1$ and reweighted K-function $K_I(t) = \pi t^2$.

The obvious method of simulating an inhomogeneous Poisson process is via IPP2, whether with fixed or randomly generated $N(A)$. In special cases, one-off algorithms can be devised. For the general case, Lewis and Shedler (1979) suggest an algorithm based on rejection sampling. In its simplest form, this consists of simulating a Poisson process on A with intensity λ_0 equal to the maximum value of $\lambda(x)$ within A, and retaining an event at x with probability $\lambda(x)/\lambda_0$.

5.5 Cox processes

The rationale behind the use of Poisson cluster processes as models for biological processes is that aggregated spatial point patterns might be generated by the clustering of groups of related events, as in Neyman's (1939) seminal paper. A second possible source of aggregation is environmental heterogeneity. Specifically, an inhomogeneous Poisson process with intensity function $\lambda(x)$ will produce apparent clusters of events in regions of relatively high intensity. The source of such environmental heterogeneity might itself be stochastic in nature. This suggests investigation of a class of 'doubly stochastic' processes formed as inhomogeneous Poisson processes with stochastic intensity functions. Such processes are called Cox processes, following their introduction in one temporal dimension by Cox (1955). Explicitly, we have:

CP1 $\{\Lambda(x)\} : x \in \mathbb{R}^2\}$ is a non-negative-valued stochastic process.

CP2 Conditional on $\{\Lambda(x) = \lambda(x) : x \in \mathbb{R}^2\}$, the events form an inhomogeneous Poisson process with intensity function $\lambda(x)$.

The point process is stationary if and only if the intensity process $\Lambda(x)$ is stationary, and similarly for isotropy. A convenient and expressive terminology is to refer to the Cox process 'driven by' $\{\Lambda(x)\}$.

First-order and second-order properties are obtained from those of the inhomogeneous Poisson process by taking expectations with respect to $\{\Lambda(x)\}$. Thus, in the stationary case, the intensity is

$$\lambda = E[\Lambda(x)].$$

Also, the conditional intensity of a pair of events at x and y, given $\{\Lambda(x)\}$, is $\Lambda(x)\Lambda(y)$, so that

$$\lambda_2(x, y) = E[\Lambda(x)\Lambda(y)].$$

In the stationary, isotropic case this can be written as

$$\lambda_2(t) = \lambda^2 + \gamma(t), \tag{5.4}$$

where

$$\gamma(t) = \text{Cov}\{\Lambda(x), \Lambda(y)\}$$

and $t = ||x - y||$. Note that, consistent with the notation introduced in Section 4.2, the covariance function $\gamma(t)$ of the intensity process is also the covariance density of the point process.

General expressions for $K(t)$ and $\text{Var}\{N(A)\}$ then follow as in (4.2) and (4.5). Note that for the typical case in which $\gamma(t)$ takes non-negative values only, (5.4) is qualitatively similar to the corresponding expression (5.3) for a Poisson cluster process. More than this, processes in the two different classes can be shown to be equivalent. To see this, let $h(\cdot)$ be a bivariate pdf and construct an intensity process $\{\Lambda(x)\}$ by defining

$$\Lambda(x) = \mu \sum_{i=1}^{\infty} h(x - X_i) \tag{5.5}$$

for some $\mu > 0$, where the X_i are the points of a Poisson process. The Cox process driven by (5.5) is also a Poisson cluster process in which PCP2 specifies a Poisson distribution with mean μ, and PCP3 specifies the pdf $h(\cdot)$. Intuitively, this is because a Poisson distribution for the number of offspring per parent corresponds to the random allocation of offspring amongst parents. The equivalence of the two processes is established formally in Bartlett (1964).

By way of illustration, Figure 5.4 shows a realization of a process of this type previously introduced in Section 5.3; we take $\mu = 4$ and a radially symmetric Gaussian $h(\cdot)$ with $\sigma = 0.05$. The process has again been conditioned to generate 100 events in the unit square and the realization shown in the left-hand panel of Figure 5.4 parallels the one shown in Figure 5.2, to which it is identical in every respect save for the increased value of σ. The larger value of σ produces a more diffuse form of aggregation which, were it to be observed in the field, might suggest environmental heterogeneity rather than clustering. Whether or not such an interpretation were sound would then depend on further biological investigation.

70   Statistical analysis of spatial point patterns

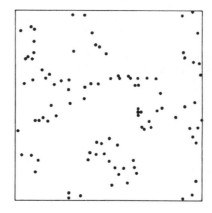

Figure 5.4. A realization of a Cox process; see text for detailed explanation.

From a statistical viewpoint, the distinction between clustering and heterogeneity can only be sustained if additional information is available, for example in the form of covariates. Note that if we were able to model the intensity surface $\Lambda(x)$ through a regression equation in measured covariates, rather than as a realization of a stochastic process, the resulting point process model would become an inhomogeneous Poisson process.

Matérn (1971) notes the difficulty of obtaining explicit expressions for the nearest neighbour distributions of a general Cox process. Conditional on the realization $\lambda(x)$ of the intensity process, the probability that there are no events within a distance t of the origin is

$$\exp\left(-\int \lambda(x)dx\right), \tag{5.6}$$

where the region of integration is the disc with centre the origin and radius t. In principle, the distribution function of the distance from an arbitrary point to the nearest event is obtained by taking the expectation of (5.6) with respect to the (infinite-dimensional) distribution of the surface $\Lambda(x)$ over a disc of radius t. In general, this is not an attractive proposition.

One relatively flexible and tractable construction for Cox processes which is not based on their duality with cluster processes is the class of log-Gaussian processes, studied for example by Møller et al. (1998). As their name implies, these are defined by taking $\Lambda(x) = \log Z(x)$, where $Z(x)$ is a Gaussian process. Second-order properties follow from known properties of log-Gaussian distributions. In particular, if $Z(x)$ is stationary with mean μ, variance σ^2 and correlation function $\rho(t)$, then $\lambda = \exp(\mu + 0.5\sigma^2)$ and $\gamma(t) = \exp\{\sigma^2 \rho(t)\}$. Figure 5.5 shows a realization of a log-Gaussian process in which $Z(x)$ has $\sigma^2 = 1$, $\mu \approx 4.8$ to give $\lambda = 200$, and $\rho(t) = \exp(-4t)$. Also shown is the corresponding realization of $\Lambda(x) = \exp\{Z(x)\}$. The asymmetric appearance of the intensity surface, with relatively sharp peaks and flatter troughs, is a characteristic feature of this class of processes.

Kingman (1977) has argued that Cox processes provide a natural framework within which to model the spatial pattern of a population of reproducing individuals. Let G_n

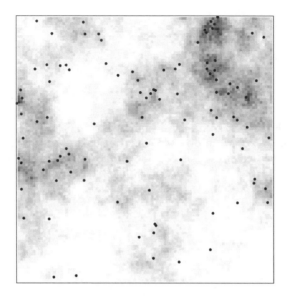

Figure 5.5. A realization of a log-Gaussian Cox process (dots) superimposed on the realization of the underlying intensity surface (grey-scale image); see text for detailed explanation.

denote a point process which determines the locations X_i of individuals in the nth generation and suppose that reproduction obeys the following rules:

1. The number of offspring of the parent individual at x_i is a Poisson random variable with mean $\mu_i = \mu_i(G_n)$.
2. The positions of offspring relative to their parents are independently distributed according to a bivariate distribution with pdf $h(\cdot)$.

Rule 2 above is identical to postulate PCP3 of a Poisson cluster process, whilst rule 1 is similar to PCP2 but allows the μ_i to depend on the configuration of parent individuals; for example, μ_i might be a function of the number of parents within some prescribed distance of x_i. The locations of the offspring define the process G_{n+1}, and so on. It follows that G_{n+1} is a Cox process with $\{\Lambda(x)\}$ defined by

$$\Lambda(x) = \sum_{i=1}^{\infty} \mu_i(G_n) h(x - x_i),$$

where the x_i are the events of the nth generation and might, for example, be determined according to the 'multi-generation' prescription discussed briefly at the end of Section 5.3.

In principle, any Cox process can be simulated by first simulating $\{\Lambda(x)\}$ on the appropriate region and then using the rejection sampling method for inhomogeneous Poisson processes as described in Section 5.4. More efficient methods can be devised for particular types of Cox process. For example, Cox processes defined by (5.5) are more efficiently simulated as Poisson cluster processes.

5.6 Simple inhibition processes

The alternatives to the Poisson process described in Sections 5.3 and 5.5 share a tendency to produce aggregated patterns. Regular patterns arise most naturally by the imposition of a minimum permissible distance, δ say, between any two events. This may simply reflect the physical size of the biological entities whose locations define the point pattern (cf. the discussion of Figure 1.3 in Section 1.1), or it may be a manifestation of more subtle effects such as competition between plants or territorial behaviour in animals. Processes of this sort which incorporate no further departure from CSR are called simple inhibition processes, a notion which can be formalized in several non-equivalent ways. As a convenient piece of terminology, we define the *packing intensity* of a simple inhibition process as

$$\tau = \lambda \pi \delta^2 / 4,$$

where λ is the intensity. Thus, τ is the proportion of the plane covered by non-overlapping discs of diameter δ, or the expected proportion of coverage for a finite region A. Notice that the maximum possible packing intensity is attained by close-packed discs whose centres form an equilateral triangular lattice with spacing δ; thus $\tau \leq \tau_{\max} = (\pi\sqrt{3})/6 \approx 0.907$.

Matérn (1960, Chapter 3) describes two types of simple inhibition process. In the first, a Poisson process of intensity ρ is thinned by the deletion of all pairs of events a distance less than δ apart. The probability that an arbitrary event survives is therefore $\exp(-\pi\rho\delta^2)$, and the intensity of the simple inhibition process is

$$\lambda = \rho \exp(-\pi\rho\delta^2). \tag{5.7}$$

The corresponding packing intensity is at most $(4e)^{-1} \approx 0.092$, or about 10% of $\tau_{\max}$. The second-order properties are conveniently expressed by

$$\lambda_2(t) = \begin{cases} 0 & : t < \delta, \\ \rho^2 \exp\{-\rho U_\delta(t)\} & : t \geq \delta, \end{cases} \tag{5.8}$$

where $U_\delta(t)$ denotes the area of the union of two discs each of radius δ and with centres a distance t apart. This follows because $\exp\{-\rho U_\delta(t)\}$ is the conditional probability that two events both survive, given that they are a distance $t \geq \delta$ apart.

In Matérn's second process, the events of a Poisson process are marked with times of birth and an event is removed if it lies within a distance δ of an 'older' event. Expressions analogous to (5.7) and (5.8) can be obtained, but only by ignoring any consideration of whether or not the older event in question has itself previously been removed. Recognition of this last aspect leads to a simple sequential inhibition process, defined on any finite region A as follows. Consider a sequence of n events X_i in A. Then the following hold:

SSI1 X_1 is uniformly distributed in A.
SSI2 Given $\{X_j = x_j, j = 1, \ldots, i-1\}$, X_i is uniformly distributed on the intersection of A with $\{y : \|y - x_j\| \geq \delta, j = 1, \ldots, i-1\}$.

Simple sequential inhibition is parameterized most naturally by its packing intensity, $\tau = n\pi\delta^2/(4A)$. Note that if too high a value of τ is prescribed, the sequential procedure may terminate prematurely. The maximum attainable packing intensity is a random variable whose distributional properties appear to be largely intractable; simulations by Tanemura (1979) suggest an expectation of about 0.547. Figure 5.6 shows the development of a realization on the unit square with $\delta = 0.08$ and $n = 25, 50, 75$ and 100, the last corresponding to $\tau \approx 0.5$. The progressive development of regularity is clear.

Packing problems arise in many different contexts. Rogers (1964) gives a mathematical introduction to the subject. Bernal (1960) was among the first to use simple inhibition processes as models in the theory of liquids. Mannion (1964) discusses the 'car-parking problem', which is simple sequential inhibition in one spatial dimension. Bartlett (1975, Chapter 3) relaxes the strict inhibition rule to replace the constant δ by a

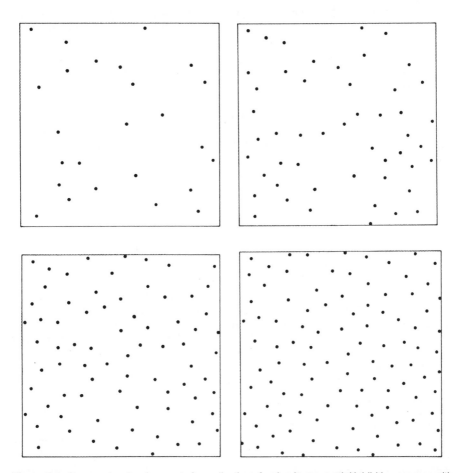

Figure 5.6. Progressive development of a realization of a simple sequential inhibition process with $\delta = 0.08$ and $n = 25$ (top left), 50 (top right), 75 (bottom left), 100 (bottom right) events on the unit square.

random variable, realized independently for each event, and uses the resulting process to model the spatial distribution of gulls' nests.

5.7 Markov point processes

Many regular patterns require a more flexible description than can be provided by a strict, simple inhibition rule. For example, competitive interactions between plants may make it unlikely, but not impossible, that two individuals can survive in close proximity to each other.

For the simple inhibition processes described in Section 5.6 it is clear that the conditional intensity of an event at a point x, given the realization of the process in the remainder of any planar region A, depends only on the existence or otherwise of an event within a distance δ of x. In other words, the process involves a form of local or Markovian dependence amongst events. For the reasons noted above, we might wish to preserve this local dependence, but introduce more flexibility into the model. This provides a motivation for the class of Markov point processes introduced by Ripley and Kelly (1977).

Markov point processes are defined on an arbitrary, but fixed, finite region A. Each process is characterized by its likelihood ratio $f(\cdot)$ with respect to a Poisson process of unit intensity. Thus, if $\mathcal{X} = \{x_1, \ldots, x_n\}$ denotes any finite set of points in A, then $f(\mathcal{X})$ indicates in an intuitive sense how much more likely is the configuration of events $\mathcal{X}$ for the particular process than for a Poisson process of unit intensity. Usually, $f(\cdot)$ is defined up to a normalizing constant which cannot be determined explicitly. Note that $f(\cdot)$ can always be factorized as a product of the form

$$f(\mathcal{X}) = \alpha \prod_{i=1}^{n} g_i(x_i) \prod_{j>i} g_{ij}(x_i, x_j) \cdots g_{12\ldots n}(x_1, x_2, \ldots, x_n). \quad (5.9)$$

We now define two points x and y in A to be *neighbours* if $||x - y|| < \rho$, where $\rho > 0$ is a prescribed value, called the *range* of the process. We further define a *clique* to be a set of mutual neighbours, and the *neighbourhood* of x to be the set of points $\{y \in A : 0 < ||x-y|| < \rho\}$. With these definitions, a point process is said to be *Markov of range ρ* if the conditional intensity at the point x, given the configuration of events in the remainder of A, depends only on the configuration in the neighbourhood of x. In this context, the conditional intensity is defined as the natural extension of the second-order conditional intensity as discussed in Section 4.2, except that the conditioning set is now an entire configuration of events in a specified region, rather than a single event at a specified location.

Ripley and Kelly (1977) establish the fundamental result that for a point process to be Markov of range ρ it is necessary that each g-function in (5.9) is identically unity unless its arguments constitute a clique; further conditions must be imposed, essentially to ensure that $f(\cdot)$ is integrable.

For a Poisson process of unit intensity, the likelihood of exactly n events in A at specified locations $x_1, \ldots, x_n$ is $\exp(-|A|)$, since $N(A)$ follows a Poisson distribution with mean $|A|$, the distribution of events given $N(A)$ is uniform on A and there are $n!$ equally likely permutations of $x_1, \ldots, x_n$. Thus, the likelihood function of a Markov point process can in principle be written as $f(\mathcal{X}) \exp(-|A|)$. In practice, this is seldom useful because the normalizing constant remains undetermined. There are close links between this formulation of Markov point processes and the celebrated Hammersley–Clifford theorem for Markov random fields (Besag, 1974).

Particular examples of Markov point processes include the Strauss process, for which

$$f(\mathcal{X}) = \alpha \beta^n \gamma^s \tag{5.10}$$

where n is the number of events in $\mathcal{X}$, s is the number of distinct pairs of neighbours, α is the normalizing constant, β reflects the intensity of the process and γ describes the interactions between neighbours. The case $\gamma = 1$ gives a Poisson process with intensity β, whilst $\gamma = 0$ gives a simple inhibition process, each realization of which is a partial realization of a Poisson process but conditioned by the requirement that no two events in the region A may be neighbours. This last process is formally different from simple sequential inhibition, but its statistical properties appear to be very similar (Ripley, 1977). Values of γ between 0 and 1 represent a form of non-strict inhibition. In the original paper, Strauss proposed (5.10) with $\gamma > 1$ as a model for clustering. Unfortunately, this results in an explosion of the process, with an infinite number of events in A. This can be seen intuitively from the form of (5.10), in which the exponent s can be of order n^2, whereas adjustment of the intensity via the parameter β can only absorb a term of order n. Kelly and Ripley (1976) establish this result formally.

If we fix n in (5.10), this results in a valid probability distribution for $\mathcal{X}$ for any non-negative γ. However, when $\gamma > 1$ the resulting patterns tend to exhibit an extreme form of clustering as the most likely configuration of events is one in which all n events form a single cluster of mutual neighbours. This is discussed in more detail in Gates and Westcott (1986).

5.7.1 Pairwise interaction point processes

The class of *pairwise interaction processes* is defined by

$$f(\mathcal{X}) = \alpha \beta^n \prod_i \prod_{j \neq i} h\{||x_i - x_j||\}, \tag{5.11}$$

where α and β are as in (5.10), $h(u)$ is non-negative for all u and the product is over all pairs of distinct points in $\mathcal{X}$ (Ripley, 1977). As the Strauss process is a special case of (5.11), it follows from the earlier discussion that some further restriction on $h(\cdot)$ is required in order to define a valid point process. A sufficient condition is that $h(\cdot)$ is bounded and $h(u) = 0$ for all u less than some $\delta > 0$; this automatically limits the number of events in any finite region A by imposing a minimum permissible distance δ between any two events. However, models which allow $h(u)$ to exceed 1 still tend to produce unrealistic patterns except in circumstances where it is natural to consider a process with a fixed number of events in a fixed, finite region of space.

To generate simulated realizations of a Markov point process the following procedure can be used. For illustrative convenience, we confine our attention to the class of pairwise interaction processes defined by (5.11), and condition each realization to produce n events in A. Let $\mathcal{X} = \{x_1, \ldots, x_{n-1}\}$ be any set of $n - 1$ events in A and consider the possible addition of an event at the point y. Under (5.11),

$$f(\mathcal{X} \cup y) = \alpha \beta^n \prod_i \prod_{j \neq i} h\{||x_i - x_j||\} \prod_{i=1}^{n-1} h\{||x_i - y||\}$$

and
$$f(\mathcal{X} \cup y)/f(\mathcal{X}) = \beta \prod_{i=1}^{n-1} h\{||x_i - y||\}. \tag{5.12}$$

Since $h(\cdot)$ is bounded, say $h(u) \leq k$, then

$$p(y) = \left[\prod_{i=1}^{n-1} h\{||x_i - y||\}\right] \bigg/ k^{n-1} \tag{5.13}$$

is a probability. Consider any set of n points in A to constitute an 'initial realization' of the process and delete one of the n points at random to produce the set $\mathcal{X}$ of (5.12). Now generate a point y distributed uniformly in A and accept y with probability $p(y)$, otherwise reject and repeat until one such point y is accepted. The process defined by alternating depletion and replacement of points according to the above prescription converges to the Markov point process defined by (5.11), but conditioned to produce n events in A (see Ripley, 1977, and Preston, 1977, for a formal justification), and is an early example of what would now be called a Markov chain Monte Carlo algorithm. The number of depletion–replacement steps needed to achieve approximate equilibrium is unknown, but it is obviously sensible to use a feasible initial realization. Ripley (1979b) gives a FORTRAN subroutine and suggests that $4n$ depletions and replacements are adequate in practice. A minor variation is to carry out the depletion–replacement steps in a systematic order, so that each 'sweep' of n depletion–replacement steps results in the repositioning of every event in the initial realization. This gives a somewhat quicker convergence by reducing the statistical dependence between realizations from successive sweeps.

Figure 5.7 shows a realization of each of three pairwise interaction processes conditioned to produce 100 events in the unit square, together with the corresponding interaction functions $h(\cdot)$. The first of these is a simple inhibition process with interaction function

$$h_1(u) = \begin{cases} 0 : u < 0.05, \\ 1 : u \geq 0.05. \end{cases}$$

The second has

$$h_2(u) = \begin{cases} 0 & : u < 0.05, \\ 20(u - 0.05) : 0.05 \leq u < 0.1, \\ 1 & : u \geq 0.1 \end{cases}$$

and the third has

$$h_3(u) = \begin{cases} 0 & : u < 0.05, \\ 3 - 40(u - 0.05) : 0.05 \leq u < 0.1, \\ 1 & : u \geq 0.1. \end{cases}$$

All of these processes impose a minimum distance of 0.05 between events. The second additionally discourages pairs of events a distance less than 0.1 apart and thereby produces a more regular pattern of events, whilst the third involves an element of attraction between events whose separation distance is between 0.05 and 0.1, giving a visual impression of aggregation. All three simulations were conditioned to generate exactly 100 events on the unit square. In most applications, it is more natural to consider

Models 77

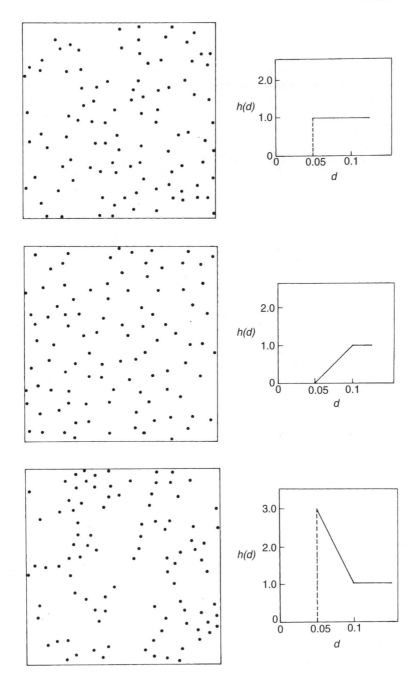

Figure 5.7. Realizations of three pairwise interaction point processes on the unit square and their corresponding interaction functions (see text for detailed explanation).

the number of events as a random variable because the study region, here the unit square, is itself a sample from a larger region on which the underlying process operates. However, for inhibitory processes with interaction function $h(u) \leq 1$ for all u, whether we treat the number of events in the study region as fixed or random does not greatly affect the statistical properties of the resulting data. In the case of partly attractive processes, for which $h(u) > 1$ for a range of values of u, this is not necessarily so. As noted earlier, processes of this kind may not even be well-defined as point processes on the plane, and when they are well-defined they tend to generate extreme forms of clustering, as discussed in Gates and Westcott (1986). Put another way, if the fixed-number prescription is used to simulate a pattern in a large region, then the partial realizations in sub-regions of a given size and shape, A say, may look very different from the corresponding realizations which would be obtained by simulating directly on A. The author's conclusion is that pairwise interaction processes should generally be used only as models for regular point patterns.

The Markov chain Monte Carlo algorithm described above can be computationally very expensive because the acceptance probability (5.13) can become extremely small. This is certainly the case when $k > 1$, but also for pairwise interaction functions which embody strong inhibitory interactions at relatively large distances.

5.7.2 More general forms of interaction

A more satisfactory construction for modelling aggregated patterns within the Markov point process framework is the area interaction process, as proposed by Baddeley and Van Lieshout (1995). In the simplest case, this process is defined by

$$f(\mathcal{X}) = \alpha \beta^n \gamma^{-A(\mathcal{X},\delta)}, \tag{5.14}$$

where $A(\mathcal{X}, \delta)$ is the area of the union of discs, each of radius δ, centred on the points of $\mathcal{X}$.

When $\gamma = 1$ this reduces to a Poisson process with intensity β; when $\gamma < 1$ or $\gamma > 1$ its realizations exhibit spatial regularity or aggregation, respectively. In contrast to the Strauss process, as defined at (5.10), the exponent of the parameter γ in (5.14) is sub-linear in n, the number of points of $\mathcal{X}$, and this prevents the process from exploding when $\gamma > 1$; instead, this case generates a stable form of spatial aggregation.

Baddeley and Møller (1989) consider a generalization of the Markov point process construction in which the neighbourhood definition for a pair of events is allowed to vary dynamically according to the configuration of other events. One of their specific examples defines two events to be neighbours if their associated Dirichlet cells share a common boundary.

For a more detailed account of these and other constructions for Markov point processes, see Van Lieshout (2000).

5.8 Other constructions

5.8.1 Lattice-based processes

Various lattice-based processes can be used to generate regular spatial point patterns. These have limited appeal as models for natural phenomena, although the equilateral triangular lattice does represent an extreme of complete regularity and as such has been used as an idealized model of territorial behaviour within a population of mobile individuals (Maynard-Smith, 1974, Chapter 12).

A more pragmatic reason for studying lattice-based processes is their relative tractability by comparison with inhibition processes. This can be useful in the assessment of proposed inferential procedures, for example to make power comparisons amongst rival tests of CSR. In this context, deterministic lattice structures were used by Persson (1964) and Holgate (1965c), randomly thinned lattices by Brown and Holgate (1974), and the superposition of a deterministic lattice and a Poisson process by Diggle (1975).

5.8.2 Thinned processes

Many biological processes involve mortality, which in some instances is a reaction to an unfavourable environment. For example, the probability that a seedling survives may vary according to the amount of nutrient available in its immediate vicinity. Thinned point processes (Brown, 1979; Stoyan, 1979) provide a possible class of models for patterns which result from spatial variation in mortality.

A thinned point process is defined by a primary point process $N_0(dx)$ and a 'thinning field' $Z(x)$, which is a stochastic process, independent of $N_0(\cdot)$, with realized values $0 \leq z(x) \leq 1$ for all x. Given realizations of $N_0(dx)$ and of $Z(x)$, the events x_i of $N_0(dx)$ are retained, independently, with respective probabilities $z(x_i)$. The corresponding realization of the thinned point process $N(dx)$ consists of the retained events of $N_0(dx)$.

The second-order properties of $N(dx)$ are obtainable from those of $N_0(dx)$ and of $Z(x)$. In particular, in the stationary, isotropic case let μ and $\gamma(t)$ denote the mean and covariance function of $Z(x)$. Then, the second-order intensity function of $N(x)$ is

$$\lambda_2(t) = \lambda_{02}(t)\{\gamma(t) + \mu^2\}, \tag{5.15}$$

where $\lambda_{02}(t)$ is the corresponding second-order intensity function of $N_0(dx)$. This follows because a pair of events of $N_0(dx)$ at locations x and y a distance t apart are both retained in the thinned process $N(dx)$ with probability $Z(x)Z(y)$. Using (4.2) and (5.15), and in an obvious notation, the K-functions of $N(dx)$ and $N_0(dx)$ are related by

$$K(t) = K_0(t) + \mu^{-2} \int_0^t \gamma(u) K_0'(u) du.$$

Note that if $\{N_0(dx)\}$ is a Poisson process, the thinned process is a Cox process. Thinned processes also provide one way of combining local interactions and stochastic environmental variation by taking $\{N_0(dx)\}$ to be a Markov point process. Figure 5.8 shows an example of a construction of this kind. The unthinned process $N_0(x)$ is a simple inhibitory process, with inhibition distance $\delta = 0.08$. To define the thinning field $Z(x)$, discs of radius 0.1 are centred on the events of a Poisson process of intensity 20. Then $Z(x) = 1$ within the union of all such discs, $Z(x) = 0$ otherwise. The resulting thinned process $N(dx)$ displays small-scale regularity due to the inhibitory interactions, together with large-scale aggregation induced by the patches where $Z(x) = 1$.

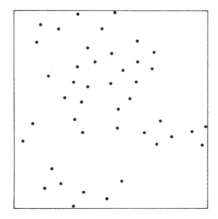

Figure 5.8. A thinning of an inhibitory pairwise interaction point process (see text for detailed explanation).

5.8.3 Superpositions

Another general construction to enrich the available range of models is to superimpose two or more component processes. For example, in Section 4.7 our analysis of the superposition of the two types of displaced amacrine cell was helpful in discriminating between the two competing scientific hypotheses concerning these data.

Provided that the component processes are independent, the second-order and nearest neighbour properties of the superposition are easily derived. In the bivariate case, let unsubscripted quantities refer to properties of the superposition, and subscripts 1 and 2 identify the corresponding properties for the component processes.

Note first that the component intensities λ_k add to give $\lambda = \lambda_1 + \lambda_2$. Now, using the result that $\lambda K(t)$ is the expected number of further events within distance t of an arbitrary event, together with independence of the component processes, we find that

$$\lambda K(t) = p\{\lambda_1 K_1(t) + \lambda_2 \pi t^2\} + (1-p)\{\lambda_2 K_2(t) + \lambda_1 \pi t^2\},$$

where $p = \lambda_1/\lambda$ is the probability that an arbitrary event is from component 1. It follows that

$$K(t) = \lambda^{-2}\{\lambda_1^2 K_1(t) + \lambda_2^2 K_2(t) + 2\lambda_1\lambda_2\pi t^2\}. \tag{5.16}$$

Similarly, using $F(\cdot)$ and $G(\cdot)$ to denote point–event and event–event nearest neighbour distribution functions, we find that

$$F(x) = 1 - \{1 - F_1(x)\}\{1 - F_2(x)\} \tag{5.17}$$

and

$$G(x) = 1 - [p\{1 - G_1(x)\}\{1 - F_2(x)\} + (1-p)\{1 - G_2(x)\}\{1 - F_1(x)\}]. \tag{5.18}$$

This construction provides a convenient illustration of how second-order properties do not completely decribe a point process. We consider the superposition of a homogeneous Poisson process and a Poisson cluster process, with respective K-functions $K_1(t) = \pi t^2$ and

$$K_2(t) = \pi t^2 + \rho^{-1} H(t), \tag{5.19}$$

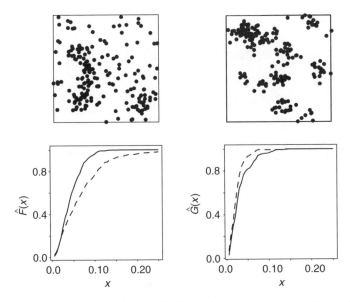

Figure 5.9. Realizations of two processes with identical second-order properties (top) and their estimated nearest neighbour distribution functions (bottom: superposition of cluster process and Poisson process (solid curve); pure cluster process (dashed curve)).

where $H(\,\cdot\,)$ is the distribution function of the distance between two offspring from the same parent. Then substitution of these expressions for $K_1(t)$ and $K_2(t)$ into (5.16) gives the K-function of the superposition as

$$K(t) = \pi t^2 + \lambda^{-2}\lambda_2^2 \rho^{-1} H(t). \qquad (5.20)$$

Note that (5.20) is of the same form as (5.19), but with $\rho^* = \lambda^2 \rho / \lambda_2^2$ replacing ρ in (5.19), showing that the superposition of a Poisson process and a Poisson cluster process is indistinguishable from a pure Poisson cluster process on the basis of its second-order properties alone. The two *are* distinguishable by their different nearest neighbour properties. The upper panels of Figure 5.9 show realizations of two such processes, which have identical intensities and K-functions but, as shown in the lower two panels of Figure 5.9, clearly different nearest neighbour properties. The difference is especially marked for the distribution function $F(\,\cdot\,)$, where the larger empty spaces apparent in the realization of the pure cluster process by comparison with the superposition process translate into stochastically larger distances from sample points to nearest events.

5.8.4 Interactions in an inhomogeneous environment

Markov point processes are used to model interactions between events. Inhomogeneous Poisson processes are used to model environmental heterogeneity. A construction which combines these two features is obtained if we replace the constant β in the definition (5.11) of a pairwise interaction process by a function of position, $\beta(x)$. Then the density for a configuration of events $\mathcal{X} = \{x_1, \ldots, x_n\}$ is given by

$$f(\mathcal{X}) = \alpha \prod_{i=1}^{n} \beta(x_i) \prod_{i \neq j} h(\|x_i - x_j\|).$$

Models of this kind are studied in Ogata and Tanemura (1986).

5.9 Multivariate models

5.9.1 Marked point processes

One general construction for multivariate models is to label each of the events of a univariate point process by a categorical variable which defines the different types of events. The categorical variable is called the *mark* variable, and the resulting process is an example of a *marked point process*.

In this context, and as discussed in Section 4.5, the simplest starting point for modelling is to assume that the marks of the different events are mutually independent and identically distributed. Under this *random labelling* hypothesis, all of the bivariate K-functions of the process are identical. More general models can be defined by allowing dependence amongst marks. For example, a *Markov random field* model for the marks would define, for each event x_i, the conditional distribution of the mark at x_i given the marks at all other events x_j. Markov random fields are very widely used in spatial statistics as models in their own right. An important early reference is Besag (1974).

5.9.2 Multivariate point processes

A different construction for multivariate models arises if we envisage a set of possibly interdependent univariate point processes realized on the same space. As discussed in Section 4.5, if the separate univariate processes are stationary and independent, the bivariate K-function between any two component processes is equal to πt^2, whatever the marginal properties of the components.

5.9.3 How should multivariate models be formulated?

Although any multivariate model can be formally defined either as a marked point process or as a multivariate point process, in practice the choice between a marked or a multivariate formulation will lead to different models. In particular, the 'benchmark' hypotheses of random labelling and independence are different, except in the special case that the component processes are homogeneous Poisson processes, in which case random labelling and independence are one and the same thing. More generally, the range of potential models for multivariate point processes is so rich that there may be limited benefit in seeking to establish a comprehensive catalogue of 'standard' models, as opposed to using the scientific context of a particular application to inform the modelling process.

As a simple example, we can contrast three hypothetical, but realistic, examples each of which formally involves a bivariate point process, or equivalently (from a formal theoretical perspective) a marked point process with binary-valued marks. In this setting, let P denote the unmarked point process and M the binary-valued mark process, and note that the joint distribution of P and M can be factorized in either of two equivalent ways, namely

$$[P, M] = [P][M|P] = [M][P|M],$$

where $[\cdot]$ is to be read as 'the distribution of' and the vertical bar denotes conditioning.

Our first hypothetical example is in the area of human epidemiology. In this case, P identifies the locations of all members of a population at risk of contracting a particular disease, and M identifies which members of the population do, in fact, contract the disease. Here, the unmarked point process P is a physically sensible construct, and it would be natural to develop a model from the factorization $[P, M] = [P][M|P]$. Furthermore, the marginal specification of $[P]$ is unlikely to be of scientific interest, and there would be no obvious value to the epidemiologist in devising an elaborate model for it. Hence, attention naturally centres on the conditional, $[M|P]$, and this is indeed the basis for the kind of case–control methodology which has been developed for applications of this kind, and which we shall review in Chapter 9.

Our second example concerns mineral exploration. Now P identifies the locations of a number of exploratory drillings, and M identifies which drillings lead to the discovery of a commercially viable grade of the mineral in question. In contrast to the epidemiological example, the mark process M now derives from an underlying binary-valued random field $\{M(x) : x \in A\}$ which exists in its own right throughout the study region A, and which is the process of scientific interest. Hence it would be natural in this context to begin by formulating a marginal model for M, within the factorization $[P, M] = [M][P|M]$. This is what is done in the branch of spatial statistics known as geostatistics (Chiles and Delfiner, 1999), although in that context it is rare to consider the joint distribution $[P, M]$ explicitly. On the contrary, it is usually assumed implicitly that P and M are independent processes, i.e. that $[P, M] = [M][P]$, although this would clearly be violated if exploratory drillings were deliberately sited at locations thought likely to yield commercially viable grades of ore.

Our third, and in this case non-hypothetical, example concerns the joint distribution of nests of two species of ant, as considered by Harkness and Isham (1983), Högmander and Särkkä (1999) and Baddeley and Turner (2000). In this case, neither factorization of $[P, M]$ seems particularly helpful. Rather than attempting to model either a point process of ants of indeterminate species, or the species of a hypothetical ant at an arbitrary location, it would be more natural to model the two component processes, P_1 and P_2 say, in their own right, along with any possible interactions between ants of the same or different species.

We have argued that multivariate models should usually be related to the needs of specific applications. Nevertheless, it may be useful to give a few examples of specific multivariate constructions, and this we shall now do.

5.9.4 Cox processes

In a *multivariate Cox process*, the component processes are mutually independent Poisson processes, conditional on the corresponding intensities, $\lambda_j(x) : j = 1, \ldots, k$, which are formed as a realization of a multivariate, non-negative-valued stochastic process, $\Lambda(x) = \{\Lambda_1(x), \ldots, \Lambda_k(x)\}$. In what follows, we specifically discuss the bivariate case, $k = 2$.

Note firstly that any dependence structure between the two components of a bivariate Cox process arises only through dependence between the processes $\{\Lambda_1(x)\}$ and

$\{\Lambda_2(x)\}$. In this sense, bivariate Cox processes provide a natural framework for modelling the joint reaction of two types of event to a stochastically heterogeneous environment, but do not incorporate any direct stochastic interactions amongst the events themselves.

Cox and Lewis (1972) adopt essentially the above definitions, but for point processes in time. Diggle and Milne (1983b) consider the extension of Cox and Lewis's work to bivariate spatial point processes, and give two explicit constructions which we shall describe later in this section.

As in the univariate case, nearest neighbour distributions are rarely tractable, but second-order properties can be expressed in terms of the corresponding properties of $\Lambda(x)$. For stationary $\Lambda(x)$, write

$$\lambda_j = E[\Lambda_j(x)] \tag{5.21}$$

and

$$\gamma_{ij}(u) = \text{Cov}\{\Lambda_i(x), \Lambda_j(y)\}, \tag{5.22}$$

where u is the distance between x and y. Then, consistent with earlier notation, λ_1 and λ_2 are also the intensities of the Cox process driven by $\{\Lambda(x)\}$. The second-order intensity functions are

$$\lambda_{ij}(u) = \gamma_{ij}(u) + \lambda_i \lambda_j \tag{5.23}$$

and (4.2) gives

$$K_{ij}(t) = \pi t^2 + 2\pi(\lambda_i \lambda_j)^{-1} \int_0^t \gamma_{ij}(u) u \, du. \tag{5.24}$$

To provide an intuitively reasonable notion of 'extreme positive correlation' within the class of bivariate Cox processes, Diggle and Milne (1983b) define a *linked* process as one for which

$$\Lambda_1(x) = \nu \Lambda_2(x),$$

for some positive constant $\nu = \lambda_1/\lambda_2$. Combining (5.21), (5.22) and (5.23), we deduce that $\lambda_{11}(u) = \nu \lambda_{12}(u) = \nu^2 \lambda_{22}(u)$, with

$$\lambda_{12}(u) = \nu\{\gamma_{22}(u) + \lambda_{22}\}.$$

This shows that the covariance structure between the component point processes is simply a scaled version of the covariance structure *within* $\{\Lambda_2(x)\}$. Substitution into (5.24) then gives

$$K_{11}(t) = K_{22}(t) = K_{12}(t) = \pi t^2 + 2\pi \lambda_2^{-2} \int_0^t \gamma_{22}(u) u \, du.$$

We emphasize that linking represents extreme positive dependence only within the class of bivariate Cox processes. Indeed, the equality of all three K-functions in a linked bivariate Cox process reminds us that such processes are examples of random labelling mechanisms which, in other contexts, correspond to a form of non-association between the component processes (cf. the discussion of the displaced amacrine cell data in Section 4.7). It is easy to construct non-Cox processes for which $K_{12}(t) > K_{jj}(t)$. For example, consider the following definition of a *linked pairs* bivariate Poisson process:

LP1 Type 1 events form a homogeneous Poisson process of intensity λ.
LP2 Each type 1 event has an associated type 2 event.

LP3 The positions of the type 2 events relative to their associated type 1 events are determined by a set of mutually independent realizations from a radially symmetric bivariate distribution.

Marginally, each component process is a homogeneous Poisson process, hence $K_{11}(t) = K_{22}(t) = \pi t^2$. However, if $H(t)$ is the distribution function of the distance between an event and its linked offspring, it is easy to show that $K_{12}(t) = \pi t^2 + \lambda^{-1} H(t)$.

To exemplify 'extreme negative correlation' Diggle and Milne (1983b) defined a *balanced* bivariate Cox process as one for which $\Lambda_1(x) + \Lambda_2(x) = \nu$, a positive constant. Note that in any such process, the superposition of the component processes is a homogeneous Poisson process.

Linked and balanced Cox processes are extreme in the sense that the corresponding pointwise correlations between $\Lambda_1(x)$ and $\Lambda_2(x)$ are 1 and -1, respectively. Intermediate levels of correlation are most easily generated within the log-Gaussian framework, i.e. where $\Lambda_j(x) = \exp\{Z_j(x)\}$ and $\{Z_1(x), Z_2(x)\}$ is a bivariate Gaussian process. Of course, whilst the bivariate Gaussian allows a flexible specification of second-order structure, it is inflexible with regard to higher-order properties.

5.9.5 Markov point processes

The formal definition of a Markov point process extends directly to multivariate processes, with essentially only notational changes. For example, a *bivariate pairwise interaction point process* requires the specification of three interaction functions, $h_{11}(\cdot)$, $h_{12}(\cdot)$ and $h_{22}(\cdot)$, rather than a single interaction function $h(\cdot)$.

We denote a bivariate configuration of points as $\{\mathcal{X}, \mathcal{Y}\}$, where $\mathcal{X} = \{x_1, \ldots, x_{n_1}\}$ and $\mathcal{Y} = \{y_1, \ldots, y_{n_2}\}$ are the configurations of type 1 and type 2 events, respectively. Then, in a bivariate pairwise interaction point process, the joint density of $(\mathcal{X}, \mathcal{Y})$ is

$$f(\mathcal{X}) = \alpha \beta_1^{n_1} \beta_2^{n_2} \prod_{i \neq j} h_{11}\{\|x_i - x_j\|\} \prod_{k \neq \ell} h_{22}\{\|y_k - y_\ell\|\} \prod_{p,q} h_{12}\{\|x_p - y_q\|\}. \quad (5.25)$$

The component processes are *independent* if $h_{12}(u) = 0$ for all u, and *randomly labelled* if $h_{11}(u) = h_{12}(u) = h_{22}(u)$ for all u.

Even very simple forms of interaction function can lead to a wide range of bivariate behaviour by varying the model parameter values. For example, consider a simple inhibitory specification in which

$$h_{ij}(u) = \begin{cases} 0 : u \leq \delta_{ij}, \\ 1 : u > \delta_{ij}. \end{cases}$$

If all three δ_{ij} are equal, the superposition of type 1 and type 2 events is a Strauss-type simple inhibition process, and the component processes are random thinnings of this. The component processes therefore exhibit a qualitatively similar, but less severe, form of regularity than does the superposition. If $\delta_{12} = 0$, the component processes are independent Strauss-type simple inhibition processes but there is no inhibition between events of opposite types and the superposition exhibits *less* regularity than do its components. Finally, if δ_{12} is large relative to δ_{11} and δ_{22} then the bivariate pattern will tend to produce segregated clumps of type 1 and type 2 events. Each component will then exhibit large-scale spatial aggregation but also, assuming that $\delta_{jj} > 0$, small-scale regularity within each segregated clump. Särkkä (1993), Baddeley and Møller (1989) and Högmander and Särkkä (1999) discuss similar examples.

6
Model-fitting using summary descriptions

Classical methods of inference for spatial point processes are hampered by the intractability of the likelihood function for most models of interest. To some extent, the difficulty has been alleviated with the development of Monte Carlo methods for calculating approximate likelihoods (Geyer, 1999), and we shall discuss the resulting methods of inference in the next chapter. Nevertheless, more *ad hoc* methods of inference, based on comparing theoretical and empirical summary descriptions, remain useful for at least two reasons: they are computationally easy, and consequently useful for rapid exploration of a range of possible models; and they provide direct, visual methods for assessing model fit.

6.1 Parameter estimation using the *K*-function

In this section, we describe a method of parameter estimation using $K(t)$ and its estimator $\hat{K}(t)$. Analogous methods using the summary description $G(y)$ or $F(x)$ could be implemented and might in some instances be necessary to allow identification of all the model parameters (cf. Section 5.8.3).

One attraction of an analysis using $\hat{K}(t)$ is that the mathematical form of $K(t)$ is known, either explicitly or as an integral, for a number of potentially useful classes of spatial point process. Plots of $\hat{K}(t)$ can therefore be used to suggest candidate models and to provide initial parameter estimates. To a limited extent this remains true in the case of less tractable models, for which $K(t)$ retains its tangible interpretation as an expectation. A glance back at Figures 5.1 and 5.2 should convince the reader that it can be extremely difficult to make reasonable guesses at parameter values merely by inspecting the data.

6.1.1 Least squares estimation

Suppose that our model incorporates a vector of parameters θ. Let $K(t;\theta)$ denote the theoretical K-function and $\hat{K}(t)$ the estimator (4.14) calculated from the data. A class of criteria to measure the discrepancy between model and data is given by

$$D(\theta) = \int_0^{t_0} w(t)[\{\hat{K}(t)\}^c - \{K(t;\theta)\}^c]^2 \, dt, \qquad (6.1)$$

where the constants t_0 and c, and the weighting function $w(t)$ are to be chosen. We then estimate θ to be the value $\hat{\theta}$ which minimizes $D(\theta)$.

An immediate question is how to choose t_0, c and $w(t)$. As noted earlier, there are good theoretical and practical reasons for not using too large a value of t_0. The power transformation c and the weighting function $w(t)$ present two opportunities to allow for the nature of the sampling fluctuations in $\hat{K}(t)$. These sampling fluctuations increase with t and so have a potentially wayward influence on the estimation of θ. By reducing the influence of large values of t we also make the precise choice of t_0 less critical. Besag (1977) pointed out that for a Poisson process the variance of $\sqrt{\hat{K}(t)}$ is approximately independent of t, so that $c = 0.5$ acts as a variance-stabilizing transformation for patterns which are not grossly different from CSR. Empirical experience with real and simulated data, some of which is reported in the remainder of this chapter, suggests that $c = 0.5$ in conjunction with $w(t) = 1$ is a reasonable choice for fitting models to regular patterns, but that for aggregated patterns something more severe, say $c = 0.25$, is usually more effective. On similarly empirical grounds we would recommend that for data on the unit square, t_0 should be no bigger than 0.25, and pro rata for different-sized study regions, but this choice can also to some extent be related to the model in question: taking t_0 small concentrates on small-scale effects, and conversely. A reasonable practical strategy is to try a few different values of t_0 and of c in order to assess the extent to which the results are sensitive to these choices.

A different strategy would be to fix $c = 1$ and use a weighting function inversely proportional to the sampling variance of $\hat{K}(t)$. Thus, for patterns which are close to Poisson, $w(t) = t^{-2}$ is a reasonable choice, although when using this approach we need to be careful to avoid problems of numerical instability near $t = 0$.

At least in principle, the sampling distribution of θ can be assessed by repeated application to simulated realizations of the fitted model. In practice, this may prove computationally expensive.

6.1.2 Illustration for simulations of a Poisson cluster process

To provide an illustration for which the correct value of θ is known, we use simulated data from a Poisson cluster process with Poisson numbers of offspring per parent and radially symmetric Gaussian dispersion of offspring relative to their parents. Using the additive property of two independent Gaussian random variables and a transformation to polar coordinates, we deduce that for this model the distribution function of the distance between two offspring from the same parent is $H_2(t) = 1 - \exp\{-t^2/(4\sigma^2)\}$. Thus, using (5.2),

$$K(t) = \pi t^2 + \rho^{-1}[1 - \exp\{-t^2/(4\sigma^2)\}], \qquad (6.2)$$

where ρ is the mean number of parents per unit area and σ is the dispersion parameter of the radially symmetric Gaussian distribution. The resulting mean squared distance of an offspring from its parent is $2\sigma^2$. In a rather loose sense, the degree of aggregation in the model increases with a reduction in the value of either ρ or σ.

For various values of $\theta = (\rho, \sigma)$ we simulated 100 replicates and estimated θ from (6.1) using $t_0 = 0.05, 0.15, 0.25$ and $c = 0.125, 0.25, 0.5$. Figure 6.1 shows the empirical sampling distribution of $\log \hat{\rho}$ and $\log \hat{\sigma}$ when $(\rho, \sigma) = (100, 0.025)$, $t_0 = 0.125$ and $c = 0.25$, with each replicate consisting of 400 events on the unit square. The strong linear relationship with approximate slope -2 suggests that the product $\rho \sigma^2$ can

88 Statistical analysis of spatial point patterns

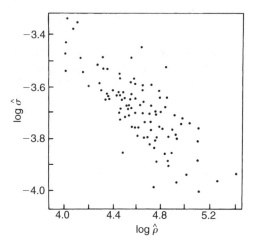

Figure 6.1. The empirical sampling distribution of (log $\hat{\rho}$, log $\hat{\sigma}$) in a Poisson cluster process (see text for detailed specification).

be estimated with much higher precision than either ρ or σ separately. An explanation is that for small $t^2/(4\sigma^2)$, a series expansion of the exponential in (6.2) gives

$$K(t) \approx \pi t^2 + t^2/(4\rho\sigma^2)$$

so that, to this degree of approximation, ρ and σ^2 are not separately identifiable. Figure 5.2 showed a partial realization of this model, but with 100 rather than 400 events on the unit square and the values of ρ and σ rescaled accordingly.

The simulation experiment confirmed that, at least for this model, using $c = 0.25$ or smaller makes the estimation procedure relatively insensitive to the choice of t_0. An exception to this general statement is that when σ is as large as or larger than t_0 estimation is, not surprisingly, very inefficient whatever value is chosen for c. In these circumstances the optimization algorithm occasionally failed to converge; the particular algorithm used in this example was the NAG (1977) subroutine E04CGF, which implements a quasi-Newton method (Gill and Murray, 1972).

6.1.3 Procedure when K(t) is unknown

When $K(t;\theta)$ cannot be evaluated either explicitly or numerically, it can be replaced in (6.1) by $\bar{K}_s(t)$, the pointwise mean of estimates $\hat{K}_i(t)$ calculated from s simulated realizations of the model. If s is large, each evaluation of $D(\theta)$ will then be computationally expensive. A sensible strategy is to start with a small value of s and use a robust minimization algorithm, such as the simplex algorithm of Nelder and Mead (1965), to find a first approximation to $\hat{\theta}$. The algorithm can then be restarted from this first approximation using a larger value of s and a more stringent stopping rule. In this context, Diggle and Gratton (1984) used a modification of the simplex algorithm in which s is automatically increased whenever the variation in $D(\theta)$ between different points θ in the simplex becomes comparable to the simulation-induced variation in repeated evaluation of $D(\theta)$ for fixed θ.

6.2 Goodness-of-fit assessment using nearest neighbour distributions

Any of the Monte Carlo tests of complete spatial randomness described in Chapter 2 can also be used to test the goodness of fit of a fully specified model, simply by simulating the appropriate model in place of CSR. Such tests are strictly invalid, and probably conservative, if parameters have been estimated from the data. To some extent, this problem can be alleviated if we use a goodness-of-fit statistic which is only loosely related to the estimation procedure (cf. Section 1.7).

We shall therefore consider two goodness-of-fit statistics based on the EDFs of nearest neighbour and point-to-nearest-event distances,

$$g_i = \int_0^\infty \{\hat{G}_i(y) - \bar{G}_i(y)\}^2 \, dy, \tag{6.3}$$

and

$$f_i = \int_0^\infty \{\hat{F}_i(x) - \bar{F}_i(x)\}^2 \, dx, \tag{6.4}$$

where $\hat{G}_1(y)$ is the EDF of nearest neighbour distance for the data, $\hat{G}_i(y) : i = 2, \ldots, s$ are the EDFs from simulations of the model,

$$\bar{G}_i(y) = (s-1)^{-1} \sum_{j \neq i} \hat{G}_j(y),$$

and similarly for $\hat{F}_i(x)$ and $\bar{F}_i(x)$.

We carried out a simulation experiment to investigate the joint sampling distribution of the attained significance levels of Monte Carlo tests based on (6.3), (6.4) and on a third set of statistics,

$$k_i = \int_0^{0.25} \left[\{\hat{K}_i(t)\}^{\frac{1}{2}} - \{\bar{K}(t)\}^{\frac{1}{2}} \right]^2 dt, \tag{6.5}$$

which are related in an obvious way to the method of parameter estimation described in Section 6.1.

The simulation experiment involved generating data as a realization of a particular model, testing the goodness of fit of that model using Monte Carlo tests based on each of (6.3), (6.4) and (6.5) and repeating the entire procedure 100 times. This produced a 100×3 matrix of attained significance levels, which we examined by sample means, variances and correlations, and by scatter-plots. Each simulated data-set consisted of $n = 100$ events on the unit square. Three different models were used, to embrace CSR, aggregation and regularity: (i) a homogeneous Poisson process; (ii) a Poisson cluster process, as in Section 6.1.2, with $(\rho, \sigma) = (25, 0.025)$; (iii) simple sequential inhibition, with $\delta = 0.08$. Realizations of these three models were shown in Figures 1.4, 5.2 and 5.6, respectively. In all cases, the sample means and variances were consistent with the theoretical values implied by a discrete uniform distribution of attained significance levels. The correlations amongst the results of the three tests are given in Table 6.1. The moderately large positive correlation between tests based on (6.3) and on (6.5) in the case of simple sequential inhibition is not surprising since the pattern of *small*

90 *Statistical analysis of spatial point patterns*

Table 6.1. Estimated correlations amongst attained significance levels for three goodness-of-fit tests

Model	Estimated correlation between tests based on		
	g_i, f_i	g_i, k_i	f_i, k_i
Poisson process	0.088	0.047	0.215
Poisson cluster process	0.048	0.268	0.004
Simple sequential inhibition	−0.077	0.467	0.001

inter-event distances is here of paramount importance. The remaining correlations are encouragingly small, and the scatter-plots showed no obvious non-linear relationships. In view of these results and remarks in Section 2.7, our preferred method of goodness-of-fit testing is to use both (6.3) and (6.4) in conjunction with inequality (2.1). This amounts to accepting the model only if neither test indicates a significant lack of fit.

6.3 Examples

6.3.1 Redwood seedlings

In Figure 1.2 we showed the locations of 62 redwood seedlings in a square of side 23 metres approximately (data extracted by Ripley, 1977, from Strauss, 1975). The methods of preliminary testing described in Chapter 2 led to emphatic rejection of CSR for these data. Ripley (1977) reached the same conclusion, but did not suggest an alternative model. Strauss (1975) used a larger set of data to fit a clustering model which was subsequently criticized by Kelly and Ripley (1976; see also Section 5.7).

Strauss noted that the apparent aggregation in these data is attributable to clustering of seedlings around stumps which are known to be present in the plot but whose positions are unknown. A Poisson cluster process is therefore plausible as a provisional model. We fit the particular model described in Section 6.1.2, in which the number of offspring per parent is Poisson and the dispersion of offspring relative to their parents follows a radially symmetric Normal distribution. We recall that for this model,

$$K(t) = \pi t^2 + \rho^{-1}[1 - \exp\{-t^2/(4\sigma^2)\}],$$

where ρ is the mean number of parents per unit area and $2\sigma^2$ the mean squared distance of an offspring from its parent.

Figure 6.2 shows a plot of $\hat{K}(t) - \pi t^2$ against t. Equating the maximum on the plot to the point $(4\sigma, \rho^{-1})$ gives initial parameter estimates $(\tilde{\rho}, \tilde{\sigma}) = (22.5, 0.040)$. Least squares estimation using (6.1) with $t_0 = 0.25$, $c = 0.25$ and $w(t) = 1$ gives estimates $(\hat{\rho}, \hat{\sigma}) = (25.6, 0.042)$. The behaviour of $\hat{K}(t)$ for $t > 0.16$ is superficially incompatible with the fitted $K(t)$, which is also shown in Figure 6.2. However, because the sampling fluctuations in $\hat{K}(t)$ increase with t, the fit proves statistically adequate. Goodness-of-fit tests based on (6.3) and (6.4) give nominal attained significance levels of 0.10 and 0.77 respectively, or, in combination, $0.10 \leq p \leq 0.20$. Graphical summaries of $\hat{G}(y)$ and $\hat{F}(x)$ for model and data are given in Figure 6.3. Note that the nearest neighbour

Model-fitting using summary descriptions 91

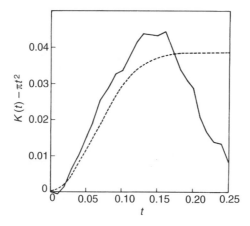

Figure 6.2. $K(t) - \pi t^2$ for the redwood seedlings: data (solid curve); fitted model (dashed curve).

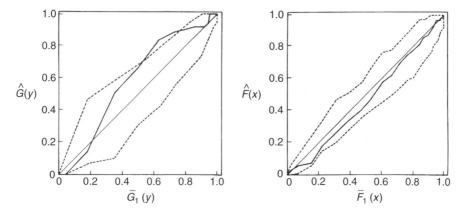

Figure 6.3. Goodness-of-fit of a Poisson cluster process to the redwood seedling data, using nearest neighbour (left) and point-to-nearest-event (right) distribution functions: data (solid curve); envelope from 99 simulations of fitted model (dashed curves).

EDF $\hat{G}(y)$ drifts briefly above the upper envelope from 99 simulations of the model, but that this does not in itself justify rejection of the model because it would imply a retrospective choice of test statistic. Figure 6.4 shows a realization of the fitted model. Both for this and for the data, visual inspection would suggest considerably fewer than the 26 or so clusters implied by the estimate $\hat{\rho} = 25.6$; the eye is a poor judge of the extent to which formally distinct clusters coalesce.

From a biological viewpoint, the fitted value of ρ implies that the mean number of mature redwoods in an area of around $500 \, \text{m}^2$ is about 26. This seems an improbably large value, although Strauss (1975) gives no indication of the age at which the previous generation was felled. Assessment of the sampling distribution of $(\hat{\rho}, \hat{\sigma})$ is therefore particularly relevant. Figure 6.5 shows the least squares estimates obtained from 100 simulated realizations of the fitted model. Note in particular the very wide range of values of $\hat{\rho}$ and the negative correlation between $\hat{\rho}$ and $\hat{\sigma}$.

92 Statistical analysis of spatial point patterns

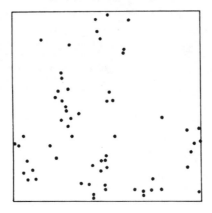

Figure 6.4. A realization of the model fitted to the redwood seedling data.

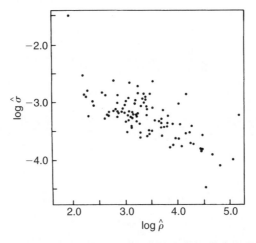

Figure 6.5. The empirical sampling distribution of (log $\hat{\rho}$, log $\hat{\sigma}$) for the model fitted to the redwood seedling data.

Diggle (1978) fitted a different Poisson cluster process to these data, in which the radially symmetric Normal dispersion of offspring was replaced by a uniform distribution over a disc of radius σ centred on the corresponding parent. This gave an equally good fit, and comparable estimates $(\hat{\rho}, \hat{\sigma})$. This example shows that it can be all too easy to fit a model to sparse, strongly aggregated data. In the present context, a model incorporating inhibition between parents might be biologically more plausible, but in the absence of specific information on this point it would be difficult to justify the fitting of a more complex model to such a small set of data.

6.3.2 Bramble canes

Hutchings (1979) describes an investigation of the spatial pattern of bramble canes in a 9 metre square plot 'staked out within a dense thicket of bramble'. Living canes were classified as newly emergent, one year old or two years old.

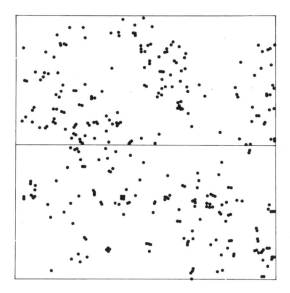

Figure 6.6. Locations of 359 newly emergent bramble canes in a 9 metre square plot (Hutchings, 1979).

We first analyse the pattern of the 359 newly emergent canes, shown in Figure 6.6. For these data, Hutchings detects aggregation using the uncorrected form of the Clark–Evans test. Although this is strictly invalid, inspection of the data does strongly suggest an aggregated pattern and this is confirmed by analysis via the EDFs of nearest neighbour and point-to-nearest-event distances.

For the remainder of the analysis we take 9 metres as the unit of measurement, split the square plot into two rectangles as indicated in Figure 6.6 and use the lower rectangle to formulate a model for the data, reserving the upper rectangle for a final check on the goodness of fit. Hutchings attributes the aggregated pattern to 'vigorous vegetative reproduction' so that, as in Section 6.1.2, we adopt a Poisson cluster process as a provisional model. Using the same model and estimation procedure as in Section 6.1.2, we obtain parameter estimates $(\hat{\rho}, \hat{\sigma}) = (68.7, 0.032)$. Figure 6.7 shows the function $\hat{K}(t) - \pi t^2$ for the data and the envelope from 19 simulations of the fitted model, together with the fitted function $K(t) - \pi t^2$. This apparently indicates a satisfactory fit, except near the origin. However, nominal attained significance levels for tests based on the nearest neighbour and point-to-nearest-event statistics (6.3) and (6.4) are 0.01 and 0.61 respectively, or, in combination, $0.01 \leq p \leq 0.02$. Figure 6.8 shows the EDF of nearest neighbour distances for the data together with the envelope from 99 simulations of the model, emphasizing the poor fit at small distances. Re-estimation of ρ and σ using $t_0 = 0.05$ rather than 0.25 in (6.1) gives $(\hat{\rho}, \hat{\sigma}) = (311.9, 0.007)$ and attained significance levels for tests based on (6.3) and (6.4) of 0.10 and 0.01 respectively; the model is again rejected, but note that the evidence for this now derives from the point-to-nearest-event distances rather than from the nearest neighbour distances.

In view of the above results, we now attempt to model the finer second-order structure apparent in Figure 6.7, by a combination of tight clustering at a small physical scale and a more diffuse form of aggregation, the latter reflecting possible environmental

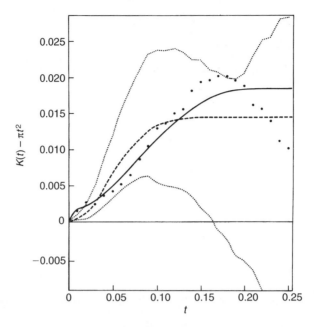

Figure 6.7. $K(t) - \pi t^2$ for newly emergent bramble canes (lower half): data (filled circles); fitted Poisson cluster process (dashed curve); envelope from 19 simulations of fitted Poisson cluster process (dotted curves); fitted four-parameter model (solid curve).

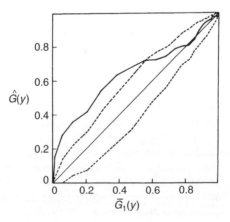

Figure 6.8. Goodness-of-fit for the Poisson cluster process model fitted to the newly emergent bramble canes (lower half), based on the nearest neighbour distribution function: data (solid curve); envelope from 99 simulations of fitted Poisson cluster process (dashed curves).

heterogeneity. Specifically, we apply a thinning field $\{Z(x)\}$ to the Poisson cluster process described previously. For $\{Z(x)\}$ we use the example of Section 5.8.2, in which discs of radius δ are centred on the events of a Poisson process of intensity λ and $Z(x) = 1$ if x is covered by at least one such disc, and $Z(x) = 0$ otherwise. According to (5.15) we need the mean and covariance function of $\{Z(x)\}$ in order to determine the second-order properties of this four-parameter model.

Note that $P\{Z(x) = 0\}$ is the probability that there are no disc centres within a distance δ of the point x and that $E[Z(x)] = P\{Z(x) = 1\} = 1 - P\{Z(x) = 0\}$. Since the number of disc centres in a region A follows a Poisson distribution with mean $\lambda |A|$, it follows that

$$E[Z(x)] = 1 - \exp(-\pi\lambda\delta^2). \tag{6.6}$$

Similarly, for two points x and y a distance u apart, $P\{Z(x) = Z(y) = 0\}$ is the probability that there are no disc centres within a distance δ of either x or y, and we deduce that

$$P\{Z(x) = Z(y) = 0\} = \begin{cases} \exp[-\lambda\{2\pi\delta^2 - A(u;\delta)\}] & : 0 \le u < 2\delta, \\ \exp(-2\pi\lambda\delta^2) & : u \ge 2\delta \end{cases}$$

where $A(u,\delta)$ is the area of intersection of two discs, each of radius δ and whose centres are a distance u apart. This result allows us to evaluate the covariance function $\gamma(u)$ of $\{Z(x)\}$ because

$$\begin{aligned} \text{Cov}\{Z(x), Z(y)\} &= \text{Cov}\{1 - Z(x), 1 - Z(y)\} \\ &= P\{Z(x) = Z(y) = 0\} - P\{Z(x) = 0\}P\{Z(y) = 0\}. \end{aligned}$$

Routine manipulation gives the covariance function as

$$\gamma(u) = \begin{cases} \exp(-2\pi\lambda\delta^2)[\exp\{\lambda A(u;\delta)\} - 1] & : 0 \le u < 2\delta, \\ 0 & : u \ge 2\delta. \end{cases} \tag{6.7}$$

Substitution of (6.6) and (6.7) into (5.15) gives $K(t)$ for our four-parameter model in a form which can easily be evaluated by numerical integration.

Least squares estimates of the model parameters, again obtained using (6.1) with $t_0 = 0.25$, $c = 0.25$ and $w(t) = 1$, are $(\hat{\rho}, \hat{\sigma}, \hat{\lambda}, \hat{\delta}) = (1013.8, 0.0026, 26.4, 0.1078)$. Figure 6.7 includes the corresponding $K(t)$, which captures both the small-scale and large-scale second-order properties of the data. Also, goodness-of-fit tests based on nearest neighbour or point-to-nearest-event distances for the data in the *upper* half of the plot give attained significance levels of 0.57 and 0.46. Figure 6.9 compares the two EDFs of the data with the corresponding envelopes from 99 simulations of the fitted model. The fit is now very good, particularly bearing in mind the fact that parameter estimation and goodness-of-fit assessment use different halves of the data.

Table 6.2 gives empirical standard errors of, and correlations amongst, the parameter estimates. These are calculated from the sample covariance matrix of parameter estimates obtained by applying the estimation procedure to 25 simulations of the fitted model. Note in particular the very large standard error for $\hat{\rho}$. Figure 6.10 shows a realization of the fitted model, which can be compared with the data in Figure 6.6. A literal interpretation of the model would be that the Poisson cluster component describes the vegetative propagation of new shoots from old canes, whilst the thinning field distinguishes between parts of the plot which can or cannot sustain healthy growth. Doubtless other models could be found which would fit the data equally well. Perhaps the only claim that should be made for this particular model is simply that it gives a tangible expression to the notion that the data incorporate two distinct scales of pattern.

We now extend the analysis to include the bivariate pattern formed by the 359 newly emergent and 385 one-year-old bramble canes. The map of the bivariate data given

96 *Statistical analysis of spatial point patterns*

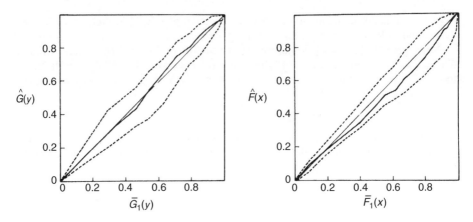

Figure 6.9. Goodness-of-fit for the four-parameter model fitted to the newly emergent bramble canes (upper half), using nearest neighbour (left) and point-to-nearest event (right) distribution functions: data (solid curve); envelope from 99 simulations of fitted model (dashed curves).

Table 6.2. Empirical standard errors of, and correlations amongst, parameter estimates for model fitted to newly emergent bramble canes

Parameter	Point estimate	Standard error	Correlation with		
			$\hat{\sigma}$	$\hat{\lambda}$	$\hat{\delta}$
ρ	1013.8	439.9	−0.34	−0.38	−0.12
σ	0.0026	0.0006		−0.15	−0.71
λ	26.4	6.6			−0.71
δ	0.1078	0.0251			

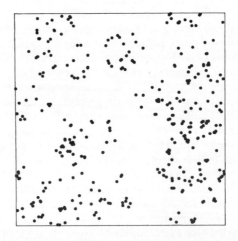

Figure 6.10. A realization of the four-parameter model fitted to the newly emergent bramble canes.

Model-fitting using summary descriptions 97

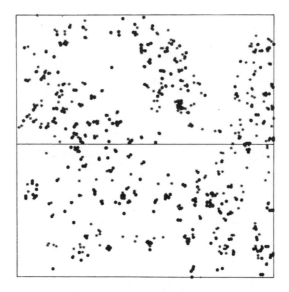

Figure 6.11. Locations of 359 newly emergent (•) and 385 one-year-old (∗) bramble canes in a 9 metre square plot (Hutchings, 1979).

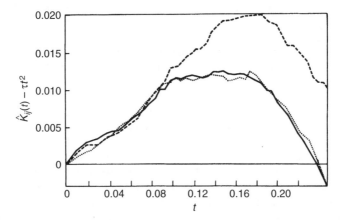

Figure 6.12. $\hat{K}_{ij}(t) - \pi t^2$ for newly emergent and one-year-old bramble canes (lower half): $K_{12}(t)$ (solid curve); $K_{11}(t)$ (dashed curve); $K_{22}(t)$ (dotted curve).

as Figure 6.11 strongly suggests positive dependence between the two component patterns. Figure 6.12 shows that the three functions $\hat{K}_{ij}(t) - \pi t^2$ for the data in the lower half of the plot are similar, at least for small t where sampling fluctuations in the $\hat{K}_{ij}(t)$ are also relatively small. In view of (4.12), this suggests random labelling as a possible model.

The four-parameter model which we fitted to the newly emergent canes is a Cox process, and within this parametric framework, random labelling of two-component

98 Statistical analysis of spatial point patterns

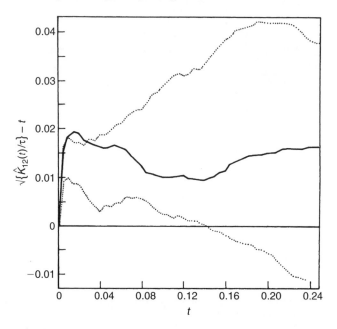

Figure 6.13. $\sqrt{\{\hat{K}_{12}(t)/\pi\}} - t$ for newly emergent and one-year-old bramble canes (upper half): data (solid curve); envelope from 99 simulations of four-parameter model (dotted curves).

Cox processes corresponds to proportionality of the corresponding driving intensities, $\Lambda_2(x) \propto \Lambda_1(x)$, i.e. a *linked* Cox process as defined in Section 5.9.4. If the two components are indeed linked in this sense, then the parameters can be re-estimated from the superposition of the newly emergent and one-year-old canes. Again using only the lower half of the plot for estimation, we obtain estimates $(\hat{\rho}, \hat{\sigma}, \hat{\lambda}, \hat{\delta}) = (1013.8, 0.0026, 26.4, 0.1137)$, virtually identical to those obtained previously except for a slightly larger value of δ; the similarity of the two sets of estimates is a natural consequence of the strong dependence between the two components.

To assess goodness of fit, we first examine second-order properties. Figure 6.13 shows $\sqrt{\{\hat{K}_{12}(t)/\pi\}} - t$ for the data in the upper half of the plot together with the envelope from 99 simulations of the fitted linked Cox process. The discrepancy for small t suggests, if anything, a stronger form of dependence than is possible within the framework of bivariate Cox processes, for which random labelling represents extreme positive dependence. Otherwise, the model fits well, in the sense that the function for the data lies about mid-way between the upper and lower envelopes. For a formal test we use the statistic

$$u = \int_0^{0.25} \left[\{\hat{K}_{12}(t)\}^{0.5} - \{\bar{K}_{12}(t)\}^{0.5} \right]^2 dt,$$

where $\bar{K}_{12}(t)$ denotes the mean from the 99 simulations, as a reasonable measure of the discrepancy between second-order properties of model and data. The test gives an attained significance level of 0.53.

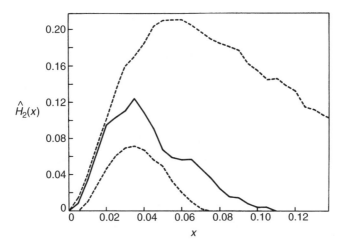

Figure 6.14. $\hat{H}_2(x)$ for newly emergent and one-year-old bramble canes (upper half): data (solid curve); envelope from 99 simulations of fitted four-parameter model (dashed curves).

As in the univariate case, it would be preferable to check the goodness of fit using a statistic which is not related to the method of parameter estimation. By analogy with the univariate case, a candidate for this task would be some kind of nearest neighbour analysis. For example, let $F_j(x)$ denote the distribution function of the distance from an arbitrary point to the nearest event of type j, and $F(x)$ the distance to the nearest event of either type. If the two component processes are independent, then

$$F(x) = 1 - \{1 - F_1(x)\}\{1 - F_2(x)\},$$

More generally, we might consider the function

$$H_2(x) = \{1 - F(x)\} - \{1 - F_1(x)\}\{1 - F_2(x)\}$$

as measuring near-neighbour dependence between two components. A positive-valued function $H_2(x)$ indicates positive dependence in the sense that neighbouring type 1 and type 2 events are then, probabilistically speaking, closer together than in the case of independent components.

Figure 6.14 shows the empirical function $\hat{H}_2(x)$ for the data in the upper half of the plot together with the envelope from 99 simulations of the fitted model. The global behaviour is again satisfactory, and there is again a hint of excessive positive dependency near the origin.

When the two-year-old canes are included in the analysis, the natural trivariate extension of the model would be to a Cox process in which all three driving intensity processes are proportional, $\Lambda_3(x) \propto \Lambda_2(x) \propto \Lambda_1(x)$. To assess the fit of this trivariate linked Cox process, Figure 6.15 shows the trivariate version of $\hat{H}_2(x)$, namely

$$\hat{H}_3(x) = \{1 - \hat{F}(x)\} - \prod_{j=1}^{3}\{1 - \hat{F}_j(x)\},$$

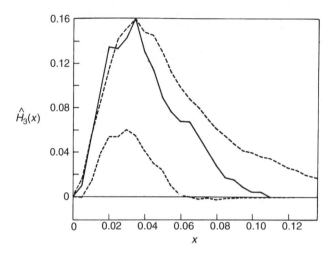

Figure 6.15. $\hat{H}_3(x)$ for newly emergent, one-year-old and two-year-old bramble canes (upper half): data (solid curve); envelope from 99 simulations of fitted four-parameter model (dashed curves).

together with the envelope from 99 simulations of the trivariate linked Cox process. Note that $\hat{H}_3(x)$ lies above the upper envelope in the range $x \leq 0.03$, or 27 cm.

There are only 79 two-year-old canes in the whole plot, as the majority of canes die after one year. A possible explanation for the failure of the trivariate linked process to fit the small-scale dependence in the data is that the surviving two-year-old canes are not a random sample from the previous year's one-year-old survivors; for example, the survivors might indirectly reflect favourable microenvironments which are not modelled adequately by the fitted Cox process.

6.4 Parameter estimation via goodness-of-fit testing

Another way of using summary descriptions in model-fitting is to exploit the duality between confidence intervals and significance tests. Suppose that we have a model indexed by a parameter vector θ, and a set of data presumed to be generated from the model but with the value of θ unknown. For any fixed value of θ we can test the goodness of fit of the model to the data. Then the set of all values of θ which are not rejected by a test at the $100\alpha\%$ level constitutes a $100(1 - \alpha)\%$ confidence region for θ. If the individual tests are Monte Carlo tests, the method involves a direct search through a discretized version of the parameter space, and is only feasible for low-dimensional θ.

6.4.1 Analysis of hamster tumour data

Figure 6.16, provided by Dr W.A. Aherne (Department of Pathology, University of Newcastle upon Tyne), shows the positions of the nuclei of 303 cells within an approximately 0.25 mm square histological section of tissue from a laboratory-induced metastasizing lymphoma in the kidney of a hamster. The diagram distinguishes two

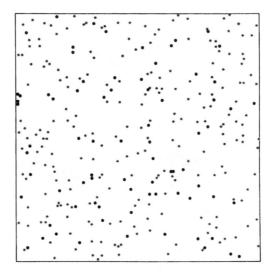

Figure 6.16. Locations of 303 cell nuclei in a hamster tumour: 77 pyknotic nuclei (•); 226 metaphase nuclei (∗).

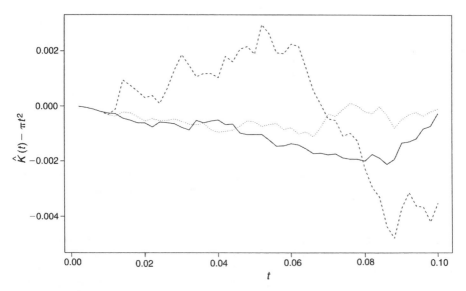

Figure 6.17. $\hat{K}_{ij}(t) - \pi t^2$ for the hamster tumour data: $K_{12}(t)$ (solid curve); $K_{11}(t)$ (dashed curve); $K_{22}(t)$ (dotted curve).

types of cells: 77 pyknotic nuclei, corresponding to dying cells, and 226 nuclei arrested in metaphase, corresponding to cells which have been 'frozen' in the act of division. The background void is occupied by much larger numbers of unrecorded, interphase cells.

Figure 6.17 summarizes the second-order properties of the bivariate pattern. These are compatible with random labelling of the two cell types, bearing in mind that the

102 *Statistical analysis of spatial point patterns*

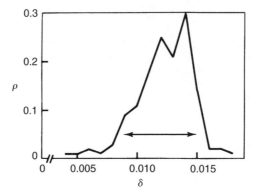

Figure 6.18. Ninety-five per cent confidence interval for the inhibition distance in the hamster tumour data.

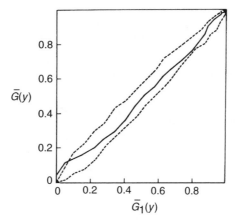

Figure 6.19. Goodness-of-fit for hamster tumour data, using the nearest neighbour distribution function: data (solid curve); envelope from 99 simulations of simple inhibition process with $\delta = 0.012$ (dashed curves).

estimate of $K_{11}(t)$ is very impressive because of the small number of events. Also, the behaviour of the three K-functions near the origin is compatible with a simple inhibition process, in which there is a minimum permissible distance δ between any two observed cells. Based on the discussion in Chapter 2, a natural goodness-of-fit statistic for a simple inhibition process would be

$$u = \int \{\hat{G}(y) - \bar{G}(y)\}^2 dy,$$

where $\hat{G}(\cdot)$ is the empirical distribution function of nearest neighbour distances for the data and $\bar{G}(\cdot)$ the corresponding average empirical distribution function from simulations of the simple inhibition process. Figure 6.18 shows the resulting p-value as a function of δ, with the implied 95% confidence interval for δ highlighted.

The particular inhibition process used in this example was a pairwise interaction process of the Strauss type, with interaction function

$$e(u) = \begin{cases} 0: & u \leq \delta, \\ 1: & u > \delta. \end{cases}$$

Figure 6.19 gives a more detailed summary of the goodness of fit when $\delta = 0.012$, corresponding to approximately 0.003 mm. The superficial lack of fit near the origin in Figure 6.19 derives from one or two observed inter-cell distances less than 0.012. Strictly, this invalidates the model, but we prefer to interpret the good overall fit in Figure 6.19 as an indication that the simple inhibition model, together with random labelling of cell types, gives a very reasonable approximate description of these data.

7
Model-fitting using likelihood-based methods

The likelihood function plays a fundamental role in both classical and Bayesian approaches to statistical inference. When more *ad hoc* methods, such as those described in Chapter 6, are used instead this is often for pragmatic reasons, of which the most obvious is that likelihood-based methods for most spatial point process models are notoriously intractable. However, this difficulty has to some extent been alleviated by recent developments in Monte Carlo methods of inference, including but not restricted to the ubiquitous Markov chain Monte Carlo methods (Gilks *et al.*, 1996).

7.1 Likelihood inference for inhomogeneous Poisson processes

An instance in which the likelihood function *is* tractable is the inhomogeneous Poisson process with intensity function $\lambda(x)$. Essentially, this is because the distribution associated with a partial realization, $\mathcal{X} = \{x_1, \ldots, x_n\}$, of this process on a finite region A can be factorized as the product of a Poisson distribution with mean $\mu = \int_A \lambda(x)dx$ for the number of events n, and a set of mutually independent locations x_i whose common distribution has density $\lambda(x)/\mu$. Hence, the log-likelihood for $\lambda(\cdot)$ based on data $\mathcal{X}$ is

$$L(\lambda) = \sum_{i=1}^{n} \log \lambda(x_i) - \int_A \lambda(x)dx. \tag{7.1}$$

In practice, this is most useful if $\lambda(x)$ can be specified through a regression model, for example a log-linear model

$$\log \lambda(x) = \sum_{j=1}^{p} \beta_j z_j(x) \tag{7.2}$$

where the $z_j(x)$ are spatially referenced explanatory variables. Cox (1972) calls this a *modulated* Poisson process.

Note that the presence of the integral term on the right-hand side of (7.1) implies that, in order to fit the regression model (7.2), we need the explanatory variables $z_j(x)$ to be measured continuously throughout the study region, A. When the $z_j(x)$ are measured only at a finite number of points within A, we need to distinguish between observed and unobserved values of the underlying continuous surfaces $z_j(x)$, and the form of the likelihood function becomes more complicated. Briefly, consider a single explanatory variable, and partition the z-surface into observed and unobserved components, $z = \{z_o, z_u\}$ say. Then, the Poisson likelihood (7.1) would apply only if we observed the 'complete' explanatory variable data z. To obtain a likelihood for the observed data, we need to specify a model for z, thereby defining the conditional distribution of z_u given z_o, and to eliminate z_u from the complete data likelihood (7.1) by integrating with respect to the conditional, $[z_u|z_o]$. How best to do this in practice is an open question. Rathbun (1996) develops an approximate approach, using geostatistical methods to interpolate from the observed z_o to the complete surface z.

For the Poisson case, Berman and Turner (1992) discuss different quadrature schemes for the integral term, and show how the model can then be fitted using standard generalized linear modelling software. Their method is implemented in the Spatstat package.

7.1.1 Fitting a trend surface to the Lansing Woods data

A trend surface is a representation of a continuously varying surface by a polynomial in its two spatial coordinates. For example, a quadratic trend surface model for the log-intensity of an inhomogeneous Poisson process would be of the form

$$\log \lambda(x) = \alpha + \beta_1 x_1 + \beta_2 x_2 + \gamma_1 x_1^2 + \gamma_2 x_2^2 + \delta x_1 x_2, \quad (7.3)$$

where x_1 and x_2 are the Cartesian coordinates of the location x. Table 7.1 summarizes the results of fitting this model, and its linear and constant sub-models, to each of the three major species groupings of the Lansing Woods data. In all three cases, formal likelihood ratio criteria would favour the quadratic over the linear or constant trend surface models. Notice, however, that the strength of the evidence in favour of the quadratic, as measured by the log-likelihood ratio, is greater for the hickories and maples than for the oaks, consistent with the relative amounts of spatial heterogeneity evident on visual inspection of the three data-sets (see Figure 2.11).

The results for the hickories and maples are shown graphically in Figure 7.1. In this example, the fitted trend surfaces capture the main features of the observed variation in spatial intensity reasonably well. Note in particular that the intensity of the hickories is relatively high where that of the maples is relatively low, and vice versa. However, as a general method, polynomial trend surface modelling is rather inflexible. In particular, when low-degree trend surfaces do not capture the essential features of the data, fitting

Table 7.1. Maximized log-likelihoods for Poisson trend surface models fitted to the Lansing Woods data

Species	Maximized log-likelihood for trend surface of degree		
	0	1	2
Hickories	3905.42	3943.57	3986.21
Maples	2694.50	2747.60	2778.30
Oaks	5419.89	5425.95	5440.18

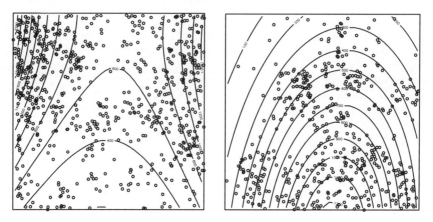

Figure 7.1. Fitted log-quadratic trend surfaces for the hickories (left) and maples (right) in Lansing Woods.

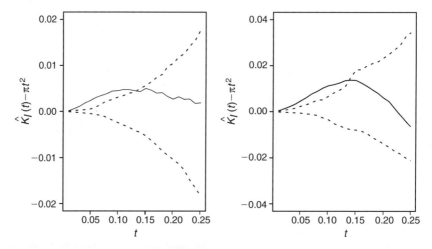

Figure 7.2. Estimates of $K_I(t) - \pi t^2$ for the hickories (left) and maples (right) in Lansing Woods: data (solid curve); upper and lower envelopes from 19 simulations of the fitted log-quadratic inhomogeneous Poisson process (dashed curves).

higher-order surfaces tends to introduce artefactual features, as is well known in the more familiar setting of polynomial regression models.

To assess the goodness of fit of the inhomogeneous Poisson process model, we use the estimated inhomogeneous K-function, $\hat{K}_I(\cdot)$ defined by (4.22), plugging in the estimated log-quadratic surface $\hat{\lambda}(\cdot)$. Figure 7.2 shows $\hat{K}_I(t) - \pi t^2$ for the hickories and for the maples, in each case with simulation envelopes from 19 simulations of the fitted inhomogeneous Poisson process conditioned to produce a fixed number of events in the unit square. For both species, there is a clear lack of fit, which could be due either to non-Poisson behaviour (specifically, small-scale aggregation) or to inadequacy of the log-quadratic model. We will revisit these data in Chapter 8, where we consider intensity estimation as a non-parametric smoothing problem.

7.2 Likelihood inference for Markov point processes

As discussed in Section 5.7, Markov point processes are defined in terms of the joint density $f(\mathcal{X})$ for a configuration of events $\mathcal{X} = \{x_1, \ldots, x_n\}$. This points to the likelihood function being an obvious tool for inference within this class. However, the normalizing constant, represented by α in equation (5.9), is generally intractable.

An early response to the intractability problem was to replace the likelihood criterion by a *pseudo-likelihood* which, for a general multivariate distribution $f(x_1, \ldots, x_n)$ is defined as the product of the *full conditionals*, leading to the criterion

$$PL = \sum_{i=1}^{n} \log f(x_i | x_j, j \neq i).$$

Besag (1975) introduced the pseudo-likelihood as a method of parameter estimation for lattice processes. Besag et al. (1982) derived a point process version by considering a pairwise interaction process as the limiting form of a binary lattice process when the lattice spacing shrinks to zero.

Subsequently, Monte Carlo methods for approximating the normalizing constant were developed, although their reliable implementation can be problematic. Partly for this reason, interest in the pseudo-likelihood method has recently been revived by Baddeley and Turner (2000). In the remainder of this chapter, we first consider the method of maximum pseudo-likelihood in more detail, before discussing Monte Carlo implementations of likelihood-based methods.

One issue which immediately arises in considering methods of inference for Markov point processes is whether or not to condition on the observed number of events, n. As discussed in Section 5.7, the distinction is not always innocuous, but is usually so for models which generate regular patterns. In developing specific estimation criteria we shall therefore take a pragmatic stance in choosing between whether to treat n as fixed or random.

7.2.1 Maximum pseudo-likelihood estimation

Consider any process defined by the joint density $f(\mathcal{X})$ for a configuration consisting of a variable number of points, $\mathcal{X} = (x_1, \ldots, x_n)$, in a spatial region A. The *conditional intensity* of a point at an arbitrary location u, given the realization $\mathcal{X}$ of the process on $A \{u\}$, is

$$\lambda(x; \mathcal{X}) = \begin{cases} f(\mathcal{X} \cup \{u\})/f(\mathcal{X}) : u \notin \mathcal{X}, \\ f(\mathcal{X})/f(\mathcal{X} - \{u\}) : u \in \mathcal{X} \end{cases} \quad (7.4)$$

and the log-pseudo-likelihood function (Besag, 1978) is

$$PL_\lambda = \sum \log \lambda(x_i; \mathcal{X}) - \int_A \lambda(u; \mathcal{X}) du. \quad (7.5)$$

For an inhomogeneous Poisson process, the conditional intensity reduces to the intensity, and the log-pseudo-likelihood (7.5) reduces to the log-likelihood (7.1).

More generally, for the class of pairwise interaction processes defined by (5.11),

$$\lambda(x_i; \mathcal{X}) = \beta \prod_{j \neq i} h(||x_i - x_j||, \phi)$$

and, for $u \notin \mathcal{X}$,

$$\lambda(u; \mathcal{X}) = \beta \prod_{i=1}^{n} h(||u - x_i||), \phi).$$

Hence, writing $p(\cdot) = \log h(\cdot)$ for convenience, the log-pseudo-likelihood function for the model parameters (β, ϕ) is

$$PL(\beta, \phi) = n \log \beta + \sum_{i=1}^{n}\sum_{j \neq i} p(||x_i - x_j||; \phi) - \beta \int_A \exp\left\{\sum_{i=1}^{n} p(||u - x_i||, \phi)\right\} du. \quad (7.6)$$

We can eliminate β from the log-pseudo-likelihood function by noting that for given $p(\cdot)$, the maximum pseudo-likelihood estimator is given explicitly by

$$\hat{\beta}_h = n \Big/ \int_A \exp\left\{\sum_{i=1}^{n} p(||u - x_i||, \phi)\right\} du. \quad (7.7)$$

Substitution of this expression back into the right-hand side of (7.6) gives the reduced log-pseudo-likelihood function,

$$PL_0(\phi) = n(\log n - 1) - n \log \int_A \exp\left\{\sum_{i=1}^{n} p(||u - x_i||, \phi)\right\} du$$

$$+ \sum_{i=1}^{n}\sum_{j \neq i} p(||x_i - x_j||; \phi). \quad (7.8)$$

This can be maximized numerically to give the maximum pseudo-likelihood estimator $\hat{\phi}$ and hence, by back-substitution into (7.7), $\hat{\beta}$.

Note in particular that the log-pseudo-likelihood does not involve the awkward normalizing constant α. Hence, maximum pseudo-likelihood estimation provides a computationally easy alternative to full maximum likelihood. Also, it can be implemented without the need for careful tuning of specialized Monte Carlo algorithms, as currently required for maximum likelihood estimation. In particular, Berman and Turner (1992) and Baddeley and Turner (2000) show how standard Poisson regression modelling software can be adapted to implement maximum pseudo-likelihood estimation for point process models including, but not restricted to, pairwise interaction point processes.

Diggle et al. (1994) have suggested an edge-corrected version of the log-pseudo-likelihood function. The rationale for this is exactly parallel to that for the edge correction described in Section 4.6 for estimating the K-function, namely that the summations of log-interaction terms on the right-hand side of (7.8) ignore potential contributions from unobserved events outside the study region A. To address this, we replace (7.8) by

$$PL^*(\beta,\phi) = n(\log n - 1) - n \log \int_A \exp\left\{\sum_{i=1}^n w(u,x_i)^{-1} p(||u - x_i||,\phi)\right\} du$$

$$+ \sum_{i=1}^n \sum_{j \neq i} w(x_i, x_j)^{-1} p(||x_i - x_j||;\phi), \tag{7.9}$$

where the weights $w(\cdot)$ are defined as in Section 4.6.1.

In practice, the integral in (7.8) or (7.9) must be evaluated numerically. In our applications, we use the simplest form of quadrature, replacing the integration by summation over a fine grid of equally spaced quadrature points to cover A.

7.2.2 Non-parametric estimation of a pairwise interaction function

In formulating pairwise interaction models for particular applications, it would be useful to have available a simple, non-parametric estimator for the interaction function $h(\cdot)$. This is needed because, in general, there is no simple algebraic relationship between $h(\cdot)$ and the already established summary descriptors based on second moment or nearest neighbour properties. Diggle et al. (1987) propose a solution which combines Fourier methods and approximations from statistical physics, but their method is somewhat elaborate and difficult to automate. A simpler solution, suggested in Baddeley and Turner (2000), is to use maximum pseudo-likelihood in conjunction with a piecewise constant specification for $h(\cdot)$, leading to a kind of indirect histogram estimator. Heikkinen and Penttinen (1999) also suggested estimating a piecewise constant $h(\cdot)$, but using more computationally demanding, Monte Carlo likelihood-based methods of estimation.

7.2.3 Fitting a pairwise interaction point process to the displaced amacrine cells

In our earlier analysis of these data, reported in Section 4.7, we concluded that the on and off cells form independent processes with very similar second-order properties, including inhibitory behaviour at small distances. In view of this, our modelling strategy will be to formulate and fit a model to the on cells only, reserving the off cells for a goodness-of-fit assessment. Also, the inhibitory behaviour at small distances, together with the absence of any obvious longer-range heterogeneity or other form of aggregation, suggests a pairwise interaction process as a reasonable candidate model.

For an initial, non-parametric estimate of the interaction function, we maximize the edge-corrected pseudo-likelihood criterion (7.9) in conjunction with a piecewise constant interaction function. Figure 7.3 shows the resulting estimate of $h(\cdot)$. Its basic shape, increasing from 0 to approximately 1 over the range of distances 0 to 0.15, is characteristic of non-strict inhibitory interaction between the points.

For the particular estimate shown in Figure 7.3 the number and width of intervals on which the function is estimated were chosen after some preliminary experimentation. The quadrature points for evaluation of the integral term in the expression for the log-pseudo-likelihood were placed on an equally spaced 24 by 15 grid.

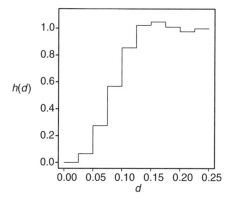

Figure 7.3. Non-parametric (step-function) estimate of the interaction function for the displaced amacrine *on* cells.

After inspection of this non-parametric estimate, we proceeded to fit a parametric model with interaction function

$$h(d) = \begin{cases} 0 : d < \delta, \\ \{(d - \delta)/(\rho - \delta)\}^\beta : \delta \le d \le \rho, \\ 1 : d > \rho. \end{cases} \quad (7.10)$$

This particular parametric form has no special scientific status, but is simply a flexible family which provides a reasonable empirical fit to the form of interaction indicated by the preliminary, non-parametric estimate. Diggle and Gratton (1984) fitted the same model, but using curve-fitting methods of the kind described in Chapter 6. Here, we use maximum pseudo-likelihood, as implemented in the Spatstat function mpl, to estimate the parameters δ, ρ and β. This involves a grid search in (δ, ρ)-space, with β optimized automatically at each value of (δ, ρ). Note that the minimum distance between any two of the *on* cells is approximately 0.032, hence the maximum pseudo-likelihood estimate of δ cannot be greater than 0.032. Again using a 24 by 15 grid of quadrature points, for each evaluation of the integral term in the log-pseudo-likelihood, we obtained estimates $\hat{\delta} = 0.020$, $\hat{\rho} = 0.12$ and $\hat{\beta} = 4.9$. Figure 7.4 compares this parametric estimate with the non-parametric estimate shown in Figure 7.3.

Figure 7.5 assesses the goodness of fit of this parametric model to the *off* cells, using nearest neighbour and point-to-nearest-event distribution functions. The fit to the point-to-nearest-event distribution is good, and a formal Monte Carlo test using the statistic (6.4) gives $p = 0.37$. In contrast, there is a clear discrepancy between data and model as judged by the nearest neighbour distribution, which shows that the model generates patterns which are more regular than the data. The corresponding Monte Carlo test using the statistic (6.3) gives $p = 0.01$.

7.2.4 Monte Carlo maximum likelihood estimation

Recent developments in likelihood-based inference for point processes focus on the use of Monte Carlo methods to circumvent problems of analytical intractability. In this section we describe an elegant method for Markov point processes which was used by

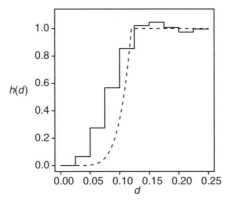

Figure 7.4. Parametric (dashed curve) and non-parametric (step-function) estimates of the interaction function for the displaced amacrine *on* cells.

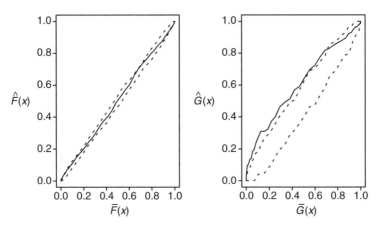

Figure 7.5. Goodness-of-fit assessment for displaced amacrine *off* cells, using point-to-nearest-event (left) and nearest neighbour (right) distribution functions: data (solid curve); envelope from 99 simulations of fitted pairwise interaction point process (dashed curves). Parameter estimation by maximum pseudo-likelihood.

Penttinen (1984), and subsequently developed in a more general context by Geyer and Thompson (1992).

For definiteness, we consider the fixed-n version of a pairwise interaction point process with interaction function $h(d, \theta)$, where d denotes distance and θ is the (possibly vector-valued) parameter to be estimated. We use $\chi = \{x_1, \ldots, x_n\}$ to denote a configuration of n events within some designated region A. Then the likelihood function for θ is

$$\ell(\theta) = \alpha(\theta) f(\chi, \theta) \qquad (7.11)$$

where

$$f(\chi) = \prod_i \prod_{j \neq i} h(||x_i - x_j||, \theta).$$

The obstacle to direct evaluation of the likelihood is the normalizing constant, $\alpha(\theta)$. However, note that for any value θ_0 in the parameter space

$$\alpha(\theta)^{-1} = \int f(\chi,\theta)d\chi$$

$$= \int f(\chi,\theta) \times \frac{\alpha(\theta_0)}{\alpha(\theta_0)} \times \frac{f(\chi,\theta_0)}{f(\chi,\theta_0)} d\chi. \qquad (7.12)$$

Now define $r(\chi,\theta,\theta_0) = f(\chi,\theta)/f(\chi,\theta_0)$ and rearrange the right-hand side of (7.12) to give

$$\alpha(\theta)^{-1} = \alpha(\theta_0)^{-1} \int r(\chi,\theta,\theta_0)\alpha(\theta_0)f(\chi,\theta_0)d\chi$$

$$= \alpha(\theta_0)^{-1} E_{\theta_0}[r(\chi,\theta,\theta_0)], \qquad (7.13)$$

where $E_{\theta_0}[\cdot]$ denotes expectation with respect to the distribution of χ when $\theta = \theta_0$. Substitution of (7.13) into (7.11) then gives

$$\ell(\theta) = \alpha(\theta_0) f(\chi,\theta) / E_{\theta_0}[r(\chi,\theta,\theta_0)]. \qquad (7.14)$$

An immediate consequence of (7.13) is that if we can find a value θ_0 for which we can both evaluate $\alpha(\theta_0)$ directly, and simulate realizations χ, then in principle we can evaluate $\alpha(\theta)$ approximately for any value of θ by using simulations, $\chi_1, \ldots, \chi_s$ say, under $\theta = \theta_0$ to obtain an empirical approximation to the expectation term, namely

$$\hat{E}_{\theta_0}(\theta) = \tau^{-1} \sum_{j=1}^{s} r(\chi_j, \theta, \theta_0).$$

Note in particular that pairwise interaction processes usually include as a special case the homogeneous Poisson process, for which $\alpha(\theta_0) = |A|^{-n}$ where $|A|$ is the area of A. However, the method may well fail unless the true value of θ is close to θ_0 because the ratio $r(\cdot)$ will be numerically unstable.

Perhaps more interestingly, (7.14) suggests a family of algorithms for evaluating an approximate maximum likelihood estimator, $\hat{\theta}$. Since θ_0 is a constant, (7.14) implies that for any θ_0, the maximum likelihood estimator $\hat{\theta}$ maximizes

$$L_{\theta_0}(\theta) = \log f(\chi,\theta) - \log E_{\theta_0}[r(\chi,\theta,\theta_0)],$$

hence an approximation to $\hat{\theta}$ can be obtained by maximizing

$$\hat{L}_{\theta_0,s}(\theta) = \log f(\chi,\theta) - \log s^{-1} \sum_{j=1}^{s} r(\chi_j,\theta,\theta_0), \qquad (7.15)$$

where $\chi_1, \ldots, \chi_s$ are simulated realizations with $\theta = \theta_0$. The remarks about the practical feasibility of using (7.13) to evaluate $\alpha(\theta)$ apply equally to (7.15). However, the method of maximum pseudo-likelihood can be used to choose a value for θ_0, which we can consider as a first approximation to the maximum likelihood estimate.

7.2.5 The displaced amacrine cells revisited

We now use the displaced amacrine cell data to illustrate the Monte Carlo maximum likelihood estimation procedure. A preliminary comment is that even with modern computing facilities, the computational load of the Monte Carlo method can inhibit its routine use in multi-parameter settings, because of the tuning required for its successful implementation in any specific application. We shall therefore explore the likelihood surface for the pairwise interaction model defined by (7.10) through a series of one-dimensional traces, varying each of the three parameters in turn.

For the initial trace, we hold δ and ρ fixed at their maximum pseudo-likelihood estimates, and vary β. We set $\beta_0 = 4.9$, equal to the maximum pseudo-likelihood estimate, and $s = 10$. The top left-hand panel of Figure 7.6 shows five replicates of the resulting Monte Carlo log-likelihood function $\hat{L}_{4.9,10}(\beta)$. Note that, necessarily, the five curves intersect at $\beta = 4.9$, but more interestingly that the maximum likelihood estimator is clearly less than the lower limit of the plotted range. The top right-hand panel of Figure 7.6 repeats the exercise, but using $\beta_0 = 2.0$ and searching over a lower range of values for β. This serves approximately to locate the maximizing value of β, but with only $s = 10$ simulations contributing to each evaluation of the approximate log-likelihood, the Monte Carlo error is substantial.

Increasing the number of simulations to $s = 100$, we obtain the result shown in the bottom left-hand panel of Figure 7.6, which suggests that for point estimation, the Monte Carlo error is acceptably small, although reliable interval estimation would

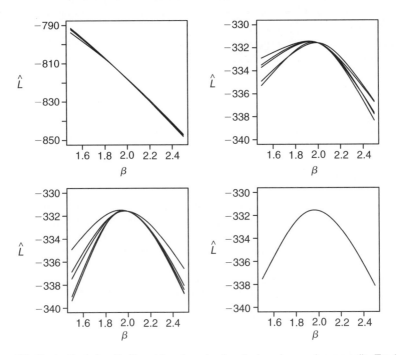

Figure 7.6. Monte Carlo log-likelihood functions for the displaced amacrine *on* cells. Top left: 5 replicates of $\hat{L}_{4.9,10}(\beta)$. Top right: 5 replicates of $\hat{L}_{2.0,10}(\beta)$. Bottom left: 5 replicates of $\hat{L}_{2.0,100}(\beta)$. Bottom right: average of the 5 replicates shown bottom left.

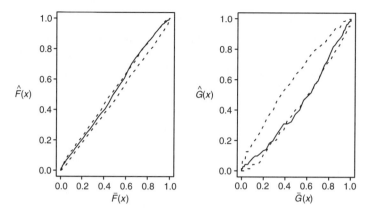

Figure 7.7. Goodness-of-fit assessment for displaced amacrine *off* cells, using point-to-nearest-event (left) and nearest neighbour (right) distribution functions: data (solid curve); envelope from 99 simulations of fitted pairwise interaction point process (dashed curves). Parameter estimation by Monte Carlo maximum likelihood.

appear to need a considerably larger value of s. Averaging over the five replicates gives the result shown in the bottom right-hand panel of Figure 7.6. The corresponding point estimate is $\hat{\beta} = 1.96$. Continuing in this way, we successively investigate the effect on the Monte Carlo likelihood of varying ρ and δ, eventually obtaining point estimates $(\hat{\delta}, \hat{\rho}, \hat{\beta}) = (0.016, 0.12, 1.96)$.

Finally, we reconsider the goodness of fit of the model using the maximum likelihood estimates in place of the maximum pseudo-likelihood estimates. In particular, the fit to the nearest neighbour distribution remains poor. However, as shown in the right-hand panel of Figure 7.7, the nature of the lack of fit to the nearest neighbour distribution is now that the model now generates patterns which are *less* regular than the data, in contrast to the result using maximum pseudo-likelihood. This indicates that the fit is very sensitive to the degree of regularity induced by the model.

7.3 Further reading

Amongst the earliest contributions to likelihood-based Monte Carlo methods of inference for spatial point processes are Ogata and Tanemura (1998, 1984) and Penttinen (1984). Recent reviews include Geyer (1999) and Møller and Waagepetersen (2002). The author's view is that the more *ad hoc* methods of estimation will continue to be useful for some time because of their ease of implementation. However, they should eventually be replaced by Monte Carlo likelihood-based methods as more efficient, reliable algorithms are developed and implemented in user-friendly software.

8
Non-parametric methods

In this chapter we discuss methods of inference which are not tied to particular parametric families of models. The material builds directly on the discussion of second-order properties in Section 4.6.

8.1 Estimating weighted integrals of the second-order intensity

Recall that one definition of the K-function of a stationary process is that

$$K(t) = 2\pi \lambda^{-2} \int_0^t \lambda_2(s) s \, ds \tag{8.1}$$

where λ and $\lambda_2(s)$ are the intensity and second-order intensity, respectively. It turns out that several non-parametric inference problems for point process data can be solved by estimating a weighted integral,

$$K_\phi(t) = 2\pi \lambda^{-2} \int_0^t \phi(s) \lambda_2(s) s \, ds, \tag{8.2}$$

for suitably defined, problem-specific functions $\phi(s)$. Before considering a specific application, we give the general result which is due to Berman and Diggle (1989).

It is convenient to re-express (8.2) as

$$K_\phi(t) = 2\pi \lambda^{-2} J(t),$$

where

$$J(t) = \int_0^t \phi(s) \lambda_2(s) s \, ds. \tag{8.3}$$

Using integration by parts to evaluate (8.3), and substituting from (8.1), we obtain

$$J(t) = \lambda^2 (2\pi)^{-1} \left(K(t)\phi(t) - \int_0^t K(s)\phi'(s) ds \right). \tag{8.4}$$

Estimation of $J(t)$ is now straightforward, because $\phi(\cdot)$ is a known function and we can substitute existing estimators for λ and for $K(t)$ into (8.4). In practice, the integration on the right-hand side of (8.4) must be carried out numerically, but this is usually straightforward and numerically more stable than would have been the case for the direct numerical evaluation of (8.3). Given a sufficiently large data-set, it would also be feasible to substitute an estimate of $\lambda_2(t)$ into (8.3) and apply numerical integration to the right-hand side of (8.3), but, for the reasons discussed in Section 4.2, we prefer the estimator $\hat{J}(t)$ based on (8.4).

8.2 Non-parametric estimation of a spatially varying intensity

Suppose that the available data are a partial realization of a Cox process, and that we wish to estimate the realization of $\Lambda(x)$, the underlying intensity process. A simple and intuitively sensible estimator would consist of counting, for each location x, the number of events of the process within a distance h of x and scaling by πh^2, the area of a disc of radius h. In practice, we shall need to adjust this simple estimator to allow for edge effects when x is close to the boundary of the study region, but we can ignore this complication for the time being. How should we choose the value of h? One way is to consider the mean square error of the resulting estimator.

Diggle (1985b) derived the mean square error of the estimator on the assumption that the underlying process is a stationary, isotropic Cox process. If the driving intensity of a Cox process has expectation λ and covariance function $\gamma(u)$, then the Cox process itself has intensity λ and second-order intensity $\lambda_2(u) = \gamma(u) - \lambda^2$. Let $N(x, h)$ denote the number of events of the Cox process within distance h of the point x. Then, temporarily ignoring edge effects, the non-parametric estimator of the realized value of $\Lambda(x)$ described above can be written as

$$\tilde{\lambda}(x) = N(x, h)/(\pi h^2). \tag{8.5}$$

We now consider the mean square error of $\tilde{\lambda}(x)$,

$$MSE(h) = E[\{\tilde{\lambda}(x) - \Lambda(x)\}^2],$$

where the expectation is with respect to the distribution of the Cox process, i.e. with respect both to $\Lambda(\cdot)$ and to the points of the process conditional on $\Lambda(\cdot)$. Stationarity implies that $MSE(h)$ does not depend on x. Taking $x = 0$ and using a standard conditioning argument, we have that

$$MSE(h) = E_\Lambda[E_N[\{N/(\pi h^2) - \Lambda(0)\}^2 | \Lambda(\cdot)]]$$
$$= E_\Lambda[\text{Var}_N\{N/(\pi h^2) | \Lambda(\cdot)\} + \{E_N[N/(\pi h^2) | \Lambda(\cdot)] - \Lambda(0)\}^2], \tag{8.6}$$

where $N = N(0, h)$. Now, conditional on $\Lambda(\cdot)$, the count $N(0, h)$ follows a Poisson distribution with both mean and variance equal to $\int \Lambda(x) dx$, where the integration is over the disc with centre 0 and radius h. Hence, (8.6) becomes

$$MSE(h) = E_\Lambda \left[\int \Lambda(x) dx / (\pi h^2)^2 + \iint \Lambda(x) \Lambda(y) dy \, dx \right.$$
$$\left. - 2 \int \Lambda(x) \Lambda(0) dx + \lambda(0)^2 \right]$$
$$= \lambda/(\pi h^2) + \iint \lambda_2(||x - y||) dy \, dx - 2 \int \lambda_2(||x||) dx + \lambda_2(0).$$

Now use the fact that $\int \lambda_2(||x||)dx = \lambda^2 K(h)$ to give

$$MSE(h) = \lambda_2(0) + \lambda\{1 - 2\lambda K(h)\}/(\pi h^2) + (\pi h^2)^{-2} \iint \lambda_2(||x - y||)dy\, dx. \quad (8.7)$$

The first term on the right-hand side of (8.7) does not depend on h, and it follows that the value of h which minimizes $MSE(h)$ also minimizes

$$M(h) = \lambda\{1 - 2\lambda K(h)\}/(\pi h^2) + (\pi h^2)^{-2} \iint \lambda_2(||x - y||)dy\, dx. \quad (8.8)$$

Now, of the two terms on the right-hand side of (8.8), one is an explicit function of $K(h)$, which can be estimated by substituting the standard estimator $\hat{K}(\cdot)$, whilst the double integral can be converted to a single integral of the form (8.2) using polar coordinates, and can therefore be estimated as described in Section 8.1.

We now consider how to deal with edge effects in the estimator $\tilde{\lambda}(x)$. Several methods of edge correction are available. The one used by Diggle (1985b) in the one-dimensional case and extended to the two-dimensional case by Berman and Diggle (1989) replaces the denominator πh^2 in (8.5) by the area of intersection of the relevant disc with the study region. Hence, if the data are observed on a region A and $B(x, h)$ denotes the disc with centre x and radius h, the edge-corrected estimator is

$$\hat{\lambda}(x) = N(x, h)/|A \cap B(x, h)|. \quad (8.9)$$

A further, and in this case largely cosmetic, refinement can be made by interpreting the estimator as a kernel estimator (Silverman, 1981). Define a kernel function $k(u)$ to be any radially symmetric, bivariate pdf (expressed in polar coordinates); thus, $k(u) \geq 0$ for all $u \geq 0$ and

$$2\pi \int_0^\infty k(u)u\, du = 1.$$

Then, $k_h(u) = h^{-2}k(u/h)$ is also a radially symmetric pdf for any $h > 0$, and a kernel estimator of a bivariate pdf $f(x)$, based on data $x_1, \ldots, x_n$, takes the form

$$\hat{f}(x) = n^{-1} \sum_{i=1}^n k_h(x - x_i).$$

The estimator $\tilde{\lambda}(x)$ can now be seen as a kernel estimator which uses the kernel function

$$k(u) = \begin{cases} (\pi u^2)^{-1} & : 0 \leq u \leq 1, \\ 0 & : u > 1. \end{cases} \quad (8.10)$$

Note, however, that the expressions given here for $\tilde{\lambda}(x)$ and $\hat{f}(x)$ differ by a factor of n, because the intensity is a mean number of events per unit area and, unlike the pdf, does not integrate to 1.

Viewed in this light, the edge-corrected estimator $\hat{\lambda}(x)$ can be written as

$$\hat{\lambda}(x) = \sum_{i=1}^n k_h(u) \bigg/ \int_A k_h(||x||)dx$$

118 *Statistical analysis of spatial point patterns*

We can then replace the uniform kernel function (8.10) with something smoother, but with an appropriately recalibrated value of h; we use the value which makes the two corresponding bivariate pdfs have equal variances.

In the original setting of non-parametric probability density estimation, Silverman (1981) points out that to obtain an estimate $\hat{f}(x)$ with good properties, the precise choice of kernel function is relatively unimportant by comparison with the choice of h. With a qualification to be noted in Chapter 9, this has also been our experience.

8.2.1 Estimating spatially varying intensities for the Lansing Woods data

Figure 8.1 shows estimates of the function $M(h)$ obtained by applying (8.8) to each of the three major species groupings of the Lansing Woods data shown originally as Figure 2.11. We suggest that a plot of $\hat{M}(h)$ should be used as a guide to the choice of h, rather than as an automatic procedure. In this respect, we emphasize two particular features. Firstly, because $\hat{M}(h)$ is an empirical quantity, multiple local minima are to be expected in the neighbourhood of the optimal value of h where $M(h)$ is relatively flat. Secondly, and as illustrated here by the plot for the oaks, near-monotonicity of $\hat{M}(h)$ is a useful indication that there is little or no evidence in the data for spatial variation in intensity.

When the underlying Cox process reduces to a homogeneous Poisson process, for which $\Lambda(x)$ is constant and $\gamma(u) = 0$ for all u, the theoretical form of $MSE(h)$ reduces to $MSE(h) = (\pi h^2)^{-1}$, which is monotone decreasing in h. The estimates shown in Figure 8.1 have been scaled so that they in fact estimate $\{MSE(h) + \lambda_2(0)\}/\lambda^2$. This implies that for a homogeneous Poisson process, $\hat{M}(h) = \to -1$ as $h \to \infty$.

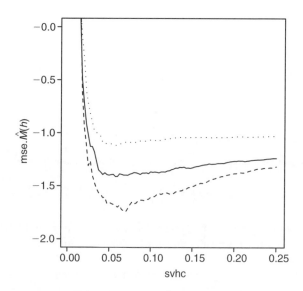

Figure 8.1. Estimates of the mean square error, $\hat{M}(h)$, of a non-parametric intensity estimator applied to each of the three major species groupings in Lansing Woods: hickories (solid curve); maples (dashed curve); oaks (dotted curve).

Non-parametric methods 119

Alternatively, $\hat{K}(t)$ can be used directly to confirm that the data are indeed spatially aggregated, and that a Cox process is a reasonable working model, before constructing an estimate of the realized intensity surface $\Lambda(x)$. Figure 8.2 shows $\hat{K}(t) - \pi t^2$ for each of the three species. The two pointwise standard error limits for a homogeneous Poisson process with the same intensity as the oaks are also shown as a dot-dashed line. This indicates that the second-order properties of the oaks are close to, albeit significantly different from, those of a homogeneous Poisson process, whereas the hickories and maples are unequivocally spatially aggregated.

We therefore interpret Figure 8.1 as follows. For both the hickories and the maples, the minimum estimated mean square error is substantially less than -1, indicating spatial variation in intensity, whereas for the oaks the estimate $\hat{M}(h)$ is approximately constant for h greater than about 0.03 and never substantially less than -1. For the maples, there is a reasonably well-defined minimum of $\hat{M}(h)$ around $h \approx 0.07$, whereas the trace of $\hat{M}(h)$ for the hickories is minimized at $h \approx 0.06$, but is then rather flat until about $h \approx 0.09$. Our preliminary conclusion is that there is substantial spatial variation in the intensity of hickories and maples in Lansing Woods, whereas the oaks show approximately constant intensity. We reach this conclusion despite the evidence in Figure 8.2 that the oaks depart significantly from complete spatial randomness. In general, we would only consider a non-parametric estimate of spatially varying intensity when there is unequivocal evidence of substantial variation and, as here, the data-set contains several hundred events or more.

Figure 8.3 show the estimates of $\lambda(x)$ obtained for the hickories and maples, using $h = 0.07$ in both cases to make the estimates directly comparable, and a quartic kernel

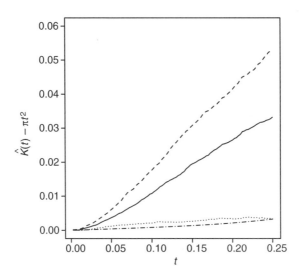

Figure 8.2. Estimates of $\hat{K}(t) - \pi t^2$ for each of the three major species groupings in Lansing Wood: hickories (solid curve); maples (dashed curve); oaks (dotted curve). Pointwise limits computed as two standard errors assuming an underlying homogeneous Poisson process are shown as the dot-dashed curve.

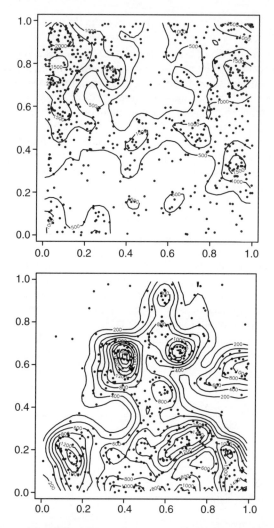

Figure 8.3. Kernel estimates of $\lambda(x)$ for the hickories (top) and maples (bottom) in Lansing Woods, using a quartic kernel with bandwidth $h = 0.07$.

function,

$$k(u) = \begin{cases} 3\pi^{-1}(1-u^2)^2 & : \ 0 \leq u \leq 1, \\ 0 & : \ u > 1. \end{cases}$$

Notice that the two estimated surfaces $\hat{\lambda}(x)$ are essentially complementary to each other, in the sense that the intensity of hickories is high where the intensity of maples is low, and vice versa, suggesting that the two species occupy distinct ecological niches. We obtained a qualitatively similar result in Section 7.1.1 using a parametric model for $\lambda(x)$. However, with the selected bandwidth $h = 0.07$, the non-parametric estimates capture more of the variation in the data, the contour lines showing considerably more

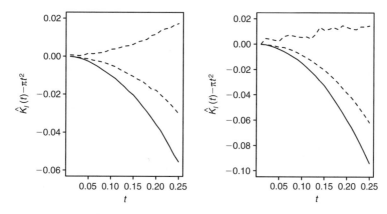

Figure 8.4. Estimates of $\hat{K}_I(t) - \pi t^2$ for the hickories (left) and maples (right) in Lansing Woods: data (solid curve); upper and lower envelopes from 19 simulations of the inhomogeneous Poisson process with intensity equal to the corresponding kernel estimate $\hat{\lambda}(\cdot)$ (dashed curves).

complicated behaviour than those of the parametric model. As noted earlier, the oaks display a pattern which is close to Poisson, implying in the present context a near-constant intensity, or an ability to exploit either of the two niches favoured by the hickories and by the maples. Of course, at a sufficiently small scale, we would expect to find competitive interactions between near-neighbouring trees, in violation of the Cox process assumption. Note, in this context, that the average area per tree in the whole forest (including a small number of miscellaneous trees not considered in this analysis) is approximately 35 square metres.

In contrast to the results for the parametric analysis of these data presented in Section 7.1, $\hat{K}_I(t)$ is significantly *less* than πt^2 when we plug-in the non-parametric estimates of $\lambda(x)$ for either the hickories or the maples. Figure 8.4 shows, for each species, $\hat{K}_I(t) - \pi t^2$ together with upper and lower envelopes from 19 simulations of an inhomogeneous Poisson process with intensity equal to the corresponding kernel estimate $\hat{\lambda}(x)$. The apparent regularity suggests small-scale inhibitory effects between neighbouring trees, but could also be a by-product of over-fitting a complicated surface $\hat{\lambda}(x)$, as noted by Baddeley *et al.* (2000). By comparison with the log-quadratic trend surface estimates obtained in Section 7.1.1, the non-parametric methodology is better able to describe subtle gradations in intensity over the study region for these data, albeit with the attendant risk that the method will find spurious features if it is used on sparse data. This underlines the importance of examining a plot of $\hat{M}(h)$ before computing the surface estimate $\hat{\lambda}(\cdot)$.

8.3 Analysing replicated spatial point patterns

Non-parametric methods of inference are also appropriate when the data consist of replicated point patterns within a designed experiment, and inference can be based on the design rather than on an assumed stochastic model. For example, in Section 4.6 we considered the problem of estimating the sampling variance of an estimator for $K(t)$, and distinguished between the situations in which the underlying process was or

122   Statistical analysis of spatial point patterns

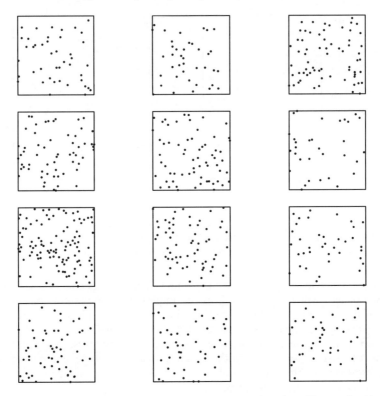

Figure 8.5. Locations of pyramidal neurons in brain tissue sections from 12 normal subjects.

was not a homogeneous Poisson process. In the second of these cases, we considered two different ways in which we might proceed, leading respectively to model-based and design-based inference. There, the design-based method used a form of pseudo-replication by dividing the study region A into sub-regions. We now consider how to analyse data with genuine replication.

Genuine replication is obtained when an observed point pattern is the result of an experiment which can be repeated under identical conditions, thus producing a sequence of patterns which are mutually independent and identically distributed. It is then natural to analyse the resulting data using the design-based approach to inference.

As a motivating example, we consider the data shown in Figure 8.5. This consists of 12 point patterns, each of which identifies the locations of pyramidal neurons within a microscopic section of brain tissue taken from the cingulate cortex (area 24, layer 2) of a human subject *post mortem* (Diggle *et al.*, 1991). The 12 subjects are presumed to be a random sample of normal brains, and it is of interest to quantify the typical spatial arrangement of pyramidal neurons, for later comparison with samples from abnormal subjects. It would be difficult to justify a stationary process model for the pattern presented by a single individual. Nevertheless, we can use the estimated K-function as a general summary measure of spatial aggregation, and the between-subject variation in estimated K-functions as the basis for inference.

8.3.1 Estimating the K-function from replicated data

Suppose that the data consist of r point patterns, each observed on a region A, and denote the ith of these by $\mathcal{X}_i = \{x_{i1}, \ldots, x_{in_i}\}$. When the patterns are strict replicates of an underlying process, the corresponding estimates of the K-function are identically distributed and a reasonable overall estimate can be obtained by simple averaging, as in the estimator $\tilde{K}(t)$ discussed briefly in Section 4.6.1. Because $K(t)$ is itself defined as a ratio, $K(t) = E(t)/\lambda$, a better strategy might be to pool separately estimates of λ and of $E(t) = \lambda K(t)$. This leads to $\hat{\lambda} = \sum n_i/(r|A|)$, which is the maximum likelihood estimator when the underlying process is a homogeneous Poisson process, and $\hat{E}(t) = \sum \hat{E}_i(t)/r$, where $\hat{E}_i(t)$ is the estimate of $E(t)$ obtained from the ith replicate. The resulting estimator for $K(t)$ is

$$\hat{K}(t) = \sum_{i=1}^{r} n_i \hat{K}_i(t) / \sum_{i=1}^{r} n_i, \tag{8.11}$$

a weighted average of the individual estimates $\hat{K}_i(t)$.

The K-function is defined so as not to depend on the underlying intensity of events. We can therefore also construct a pooled estimate without assuming a common intensity across all replicates; this presumes that the hypothesis of a common K-function and varying intensity between replicates is scientifically plausible, as would be the case if the 'replicates' were differentially thinned versions of a common underlying process. However, in this case we would again argue that the weighted average (8.11) is an appropriate estimator, since the dominant term in the variance of the component $\hat{K}_i(t)$ is of order n_i^{-1}.

For a design-based assessment of the sampling variance of $\hat{K}(t)$, we use a simple method based on the bootstrap (Efron and Tibshirani, 1993). Define *residual K-functions*,

$$R_i(t) = n_i^{0.5} \{\hat{K}_i(t) - \hat{K}(t)\} : i = 1, \ldots, r. \tag{8.12}$$

To a first approximation, the $R_i(t)$ are exchangeable under the assumption that the underlying processes may differ in their intensities, but are otherwise identical. We then construct a bootstrap sample of K-functions as

$$K_i^*(t) = \hat{K}(t) + n_i^{-0.5} R_i^*(t) : i = 1, \ldots, r,$$

where the $R_i^*(\cdot)$ are sampled at random with replacement from the set $\{R_1(\cdot), \ldots, R_r(\cdot)\}$, and compute a resampled $\hat{K}(t)$ as

$$\hat{K}^*(t) = \sum_{i=1}^{r} n_i \hat{K}_i^*(t) / \sum_{i=1}^{r} n_i.$$

Repeating this whole procedure, say s times, we then take the sample variance of the s values of $\hat{K}^*(t)$ as the bootstrap approximation to the sampling variance of $\hat{K}(t)$. Note that, because the whole of each residual K-function is resampled, the procedure gives a bootstrap estimate of the variance matrix of the vector of values of $\hat{K}(t)$ for the different values of t under consideration, if required.

Figure 8.6 shows the estimate $\hat{K}(t) - \pi t^2$ for the data in Figure 8.5, together with plus and minus two bootstrap standard error limits, computed from $s = 1000$ resamples.

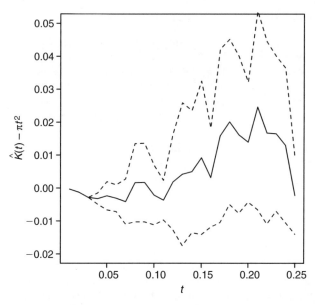

Figure 8.6. Pooled estimate $\hat{K}(t) - \pi t^2$ from 12 control subjects, with bootstrapped plus and minus two pointwise standard error limits.

Using a larger number of resamples did not materially change the bootstrap variance estimates. All of the original estimated K-functions, and hence necessarily all of their bootstrap resampled counterparts, have $\hat{K}(t) = 0$ for small distances $t < 0.03$ approximately, suggestive of small-scale regularity. At larger distances, the rapidly increasing width of the bootstrap standard error limits renders non-significant any further departure from an underlying $K(t) = \pi t^2$.

8.3.2 Between-group comparisons in designed experiments

We now extend our motivating example to include data from two further experimental groups, consisting of post-mortem samples from subjects previously diagnosed as schizo-affective or schizophrenic. These data are shown in Figures 8.7 and 8.8. One of the patterns from the schizophrenic group has only two pyramidal neurons and we shall ignore it in the subsequent analysis.

Preliminary analysis of the counts n_i, using a log-linear Poisson regression model, suggested that the intensity of events varied significantly between groups. The observed mean numbers of cells per pattern in the three groups were 54.6 for the controls, 45.1 for the schizo-affectives and 37.4 (excluding the pattern with only two cells) for the schizophrenics. The likelihood ratio statistic to test for equality of the three underlying population means within the Poisson log-linear model was 33.3 on 2 degrees of freedom. There is no formal justification for assuming Poisson counts in this context, but unless the individual patterns are spatially aggregated, a Poisson approximation should be conservative (McCullagh and Nelder, 1989). Recall that the estimator $\hat{K}(t)$ remains valid when the underlying intensities vary between replicates, and therefore also when the intensities vary between groups. Figure 8.9 shows the resulting estimates

Non-parametric methods

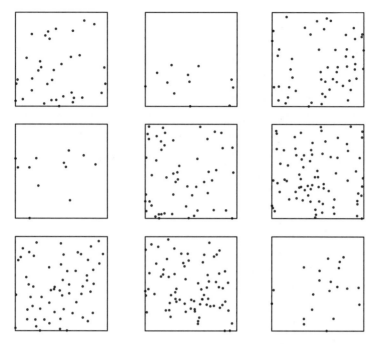

Figure 8.7. Locations of pyramidal neurons in brain tissue sections from 9 schizo-affective subjects.

of $K(t) - \pi t^2$ for the schizo-affectives and for the schizophrenics, together with pointwise limits constructed as plus and minus two bootstrap standard errors. Note that a common scale has been used for all three groups. Visual inspection of Figures 8.6 and 8.9 suggests that all three groups show small-scale inhibitory behaviour, as is to be expected in most microanatomical applications where the events represent reference locations for finite-sized objects. However, the groups appear to differ in their larger-scale behaviour; specifically, the schizo-affectives alone show apparently significant spatial aggregation. We now consider how to convert this visual assessment into a formal inference.

Let n_{ij} denote the number of events for the jth subject within the ith experimental group, and $\hat{K}_{ij}(t)$ the corresponding estimated K-function. Define $\hat{K}_i(t)$ to be the estimate (8.11) calculated from the r_i subjects in the ith group, and $\hat{K}_0(t)$ a weighted average of the $\hat{K}_i(t)$ with weights proportional to the total numbers of events, $n_i = \sum_{j=1}^{r_i} n_{ij}$, in the three groups. Now let $K_i(t)$ denote the expectation of $\hat{K}_{ij}(t)$ under repeated sampling. The null hypothesis is that this is the same in all three groups, hence $K_i(t) = K(t)$. Then the $\hat{K}_i(t)$ estimate the corresponding $K_i(t)$, whilst $\hat{K}_0(t)$ estimates $K(t)$ under the null hypothesis that $K_i(t) = K(t)$ for all i.

To test the hypothesis that $K_i(t) = K(t)$, a statistic loosely analogous to the between-treatment sum of squares in a classical analysis of variance is

$$BTSS = \sum_{i=1}^{3} n_i \int_0^{t_0} w(t)\{\hat{K}_i(t) - \hat{K}_0(t)\}^2 \, dt. \qquad (8.13)$$

126   *Statistical analysis of spatial point patterns*

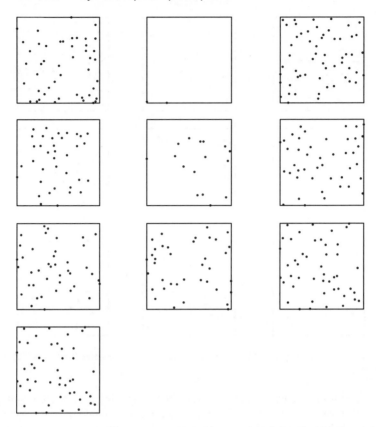

Figure 8.8. Locations of pyramidal neurons in brain tissue sections from 10 schizophrenic subjects.

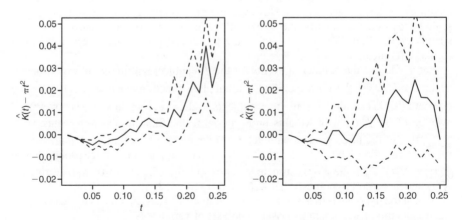

Figure 8.9. Pooled estimates $\hat{K}(t) - \pi t^2$ from 9 schizo-affective subjects (left) and from 9 schizophrenic subjects (right), with bootstrapped plus and minus two pointwise standard error limits.

The null sampling distribution of BTSS is intractable, but for a design-based inference we can again use a resampling method. For the jth subject within the ith group, define the *residual K-function*,

$$R_{ij}(t) = n_{ij}^{0.5}\{\hat{K}_{ij}(t) - \hat{K}_i(t)\}. \tag{8.14}$$

The $R_{ij}(t)$ are, to a first approximation, exchangeable under the null or alternative hypotheses. Hence, if $R_{ij}^*(t) : j = 1, \ldots, r_i : i = 1, 2, 3$ are obtained from the original $R_{ij}(t)$ by resampling, we can construct a set of resampled K-functions under the null hypothesis as

$$\hat{K}_{ij}^*(t) = \hat{K}_0(t) + n_{ij}^{-0.5} R_{ij}^*(t). \tag{8.15}$$

For an approximate test, we then compare the observed value, $BTSS_1$ say, with values $BTSS_k : k = 2, \ldots, s$ from independent sets of resampled $K_{ij}^*(t)$.

We applied the bootstrap procedure with $t_0 = 0.25$, $w(t) = t^{-2}$ and 1000 resamples. Note that in this context, each resample is a complete set of 30 estimated K-functions in three groups, but generated under the null hypothesis that the three underlying group-mean K-functions are equal. The resulting bootstrap p-value is 0.253, giving no reason formally to reject the null hypothesis.

Diggle *et al.* (1991) used an unweighted version of the test statistic (8.13) in conjunction with a square root transformation of $\hat{K}(t)$. They also used random permutations of the residual K-functions, i.e. resampling without replacement, rather than the bootstrap resampling with replacement implemented here.

8.3.3 Parametric or non-parametric methods?

We have argued that for the application described here, parametric modelling assumptions would be hard to justify, and a non-parametric, design-based approach seems natural. Of course, in this context an estimated K-function is just one of many possible *ad hoc* summary statistics which could be calculated from each pattern. It is a reasonable choice when there is scientific interest in the degree of spatial aggregation or regularity in the component patterns and in the extent to which this varies between groups of subjects. For more specific alternative hypotheses, other summary statistics may be preferable.

In particular, in some applications it may be reasonable to fit a parametric model using likelihood-based methods as described in Chapter 7. An immediate benefit is that the information from independent replicates can then be combined objectively, by adding the corresponding log-likelihood (or log-pseudo-likelihood) contributions. The corresponding cost is the reliance on additional assumptions, i.e. the correctness of the assumed model. An intermediate strategy is to use likelihood-based methods to estimate model parameters as summary statistics for each replicate, but to continue to use the randomization distribution induced by the study design as the basis for inference. Diggle, Mateu and Clough (2000) report some empirical comparisons of the parametric and non-parametric approaches, which confirm that the parametric approach is more powerful when its underlying assumptions are satisfied, but correspondingly less robust to departures from the assumptions.

9
Point process methods in spatial epidemiology

9.1 Introduction

Epidemiology is concerned with the study of patterns of disease incidence and prevalence in human populations, and with the identification and estimation of risk factors associated with particular diseases. Until relatively recently, epidemiological studies only considered spatial risk factors at a relatively coarse geographical scale, for example comparing estimates of disease risk in different countries, or otherwise defined administrative regions. The advent of relatively precise post-code systems, together with the inclusion of post-coded information on place of birth, residence or death in disease registers and in census data, has led to the possibility of considering much more detailed spatial effects on disease risk. For example, the UK post-code system is notionally accurate to an order of magnitude of tens of metres in urban areas, where each post-code typically identifies a single street. As a result, the last ten years or so have seen the development of statistical methods which apply the ideas of spatial point processes to epidemiological data, specifically to the study of the observed pattern of disease in relation to possible environmental risk factors. In epidemiology, studies of this kind are often called *individual-level* studies. Studies which compare disease rates between different populations are usually called *area-level studies* or, somewhat quaintly, *ecological studies*.

Using point process methods to model the spatial pattern of disease is not an uncontroversial thing to do. At one level, it is obvious that allocating a person to a unique spatial location is no more than a convenient mathematical fiction. Even discounting long-term migration effects, most people move from place to place as they go about their daily business. Nevertheless, in the absence of direct, person-specific environmental dose monitoring, the location in which a person lives or works, according to context, may be the best available surrogate for the microenvironment to which they are principally exposed.

Another limitation of individual-level studies is that relevant collateral information, for example on demographic or socioeconomic variables, is often only available on a larger spatial scale, for example at the level of counties or other administratively defined units. Against this, a powerful counter-argument is the well-known phenomenon of *ecological bias*, sometimes also called the *ecological fallacy* (see, for example, Greenland and Morgenstern, 1989). This refers to the fact that effects of risk factors averaged over

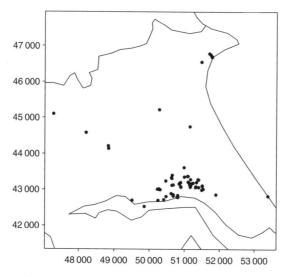

Figure 9.1. Residential locations at birth of 62 cases of childhood leukaemia in North Humberside, UK (Cuzick and Edwards, 1990). Axis labels are grid reference northings and eastings.

populations may differ, perhaps even qualitatively, from the corresponding effects at the individual level. An early example is discussed in Selvin (1958).

Our aim in this chapter is to show how spatial point process methodology can be applied to several common problems in environmental epidemiology. We do not attempt to discuss the wider role which spatial statistical methods, including but not restricted to point process methods, can play in epidemiology. For a recent overview from this wider perspective, see for example Elliott *et al.* (2000).

The starting point for an individual-level analysis is a set of data giving the locations of all known *cases* of a particular disease within a designated study region A over a defined time-period. For example, Figure 9.1, based on data from Cuzick and Edwards (1990), shows the residential locations of 62 cases of childhood leukaemia diagnosed in the North Humberside region of the UK, in the years 1974 to 1982.

A feature of all data of this kind is that the spatial distribution of cases must to some extent reflect the spatial distribution of the underlying population. In Figure 9.1, the most obvious feature of the map is therefore the concentration of cases in the city of Hull. Usually, patterns attributable solely to population distribution are not of interest, and it is therefore necessary to compare the case map with a map of *controls* sampled from the underlying population at risk. The simplest case–control design is the completely randomized design, in which the controls are an independent random sample from the underlying population. Figure 9.2 shows a map of 143 controls sampled at random from the birth register for the North Humberside region over the years 1974 to 1982. Note the superficial similarity to Figure 9.1, in the sense that the pattern broadly follow that of the underlying population at risk. The polygon superimposed on Figure 9.2 is a crude approximation to the boundary of the North Humberside region, and will be used as such in the analysis reported in Section 9.2 below.

More sophisticated case–control designs involve stratification or matching; for example, a sample of controls may be constrained to show the same sex ratio as the set

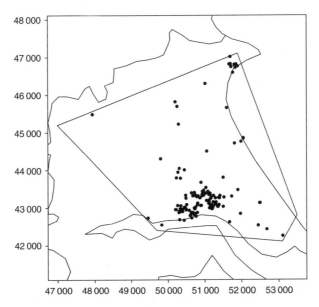

Figure 9.2. Residential locations of 143 controls in North Humberside, sampled at random from the birth register (Cuzick and Edwards, 1990). Axis labels are grid reference northings and eastings.

of cases (*stratification* by sex), or controls may be paired with individual cases of the same age (*matching* by age). In what follows, we shall initially assume a completely randomized design. In Section 9.5 we discuss briefly how the associated statistical methods can be extended to cover stratified or matched designs. For a general discussion of the arguments for and against matching in case–control study designs, we refer the reader to the standard epidemiological text by Breslow and Day (1980).

We shall discuss three classes of problem: investigation of spatial clustering of cases; non-parametric estimation of spatial variation in disease risk; and parametric modelling of elevation in risk near a point source of environmental pollution.

9.2 Spatial clustering

By *spatial clustering* we mean a general tendency for cases to occur more closely together than would be compatible with random sampling from the population at risk. We emphasize that this is a description of the underlying disease process, rather than of the study region itself. The implication of clustering is that the conditional intensity of cases at an arbitrary location y, given a case at a nearby location x, is greater than the unconditional intensity of cases at y, i.e. clustering involves a form of dependence between cases.

Under the null hypothesis of no clustering, cases form a spatially random sample from the underlying population. By design, controls necessarily form a spatially random sample from this same population. Hence, no spatial clustering is equivalent to random labelling of the bivariate point process of cases and controls, and under this hypothesis the function

$$D(t) = K_{11}(t) - K_{22}(t) \tag{9.1}$$

is identically zero. More generally, $K_{22}(t)$ measures the degree of spatial aggregation of the population at risk, whereas $K_{11}(t)$ measures the cumulative effect of this same spatial aggregation together with any additional effect of clustering. Hence, $D(t)$ measures spatial clustering in the same way that $K(t) - \pi t^2$ measures the degree of spatial aggregation in a univariate process. We shall therefore develop a statistic to test the hypothesis of no clustering based on the corresponding empirical function,

$$\hat{D}(t) = \hat{K}_{11}(t) - \hat{K}_{22}(t),$$

where the case and control K-functions are estimated using (4.14).

In order to construct a formal test, we need to evaluate the null sampling distribution of $\hat{D}(t)$. In particular, although $D(t)$ itself is motivated by the theory of stationary spatial point processes, it would be inappropriate to assume stationarity in the present context because of the spatial heterogeneity inherent in human settlement patterns. We therefore turn to design-based inference, and use the sampling distribution of $\hat{D}(t)$ induced by the random labelling process conditional on the observed superposition of cases and controls.

Diggle and Chetwynd (1991) use combinatorial arguments to show that under random labelling of cases and controls, $E[\hat{D}(t)] = 0$ exactly. They also derive an explicit, albeit cumbersome, formula for the covariance $\text{Cov}\{\hat{D}(t), \hat{D}(s)\}$. Based on these results, Diggle and Chetwynd (1991) suggest the test statistic

$$D = \int_0^{t_0} w(t)\hat{D}(t)dt, \tag{9.2}$$

where $w(t) = \text{Var}\{\hat{D}(t)\}^{-0.5}$. In applications, this requires a choice to be made for the upper limit of integration t_0. Our view is that this choice should be context-dependent, although (9.2) implicitly downweights large distances because the randomization variance of $\hat{D}(t)$ increases with t, and this makes the choice less critical than it would otherwise be.

For an exact, Monte Carlo test, we compare the observed value of D with values computed after independent random relabellings of the cases and controls. A normal approximation is also available if required, using the known form for the covariance structure of $\hat{D}(\cdot)$.

9.2.1 Analysis of the North Humberside childhood leukaemia data

Figure 9.3 shows the resulting analysis of the North Humberside childhood leukaemia data. The unit of distance is 100 km. At distances of the order of several hundred metres the empirical function $\hat{D}(t)$ drifts close to or beyond the upper limit of two pointwise standard errors under the null hypothesis of no clustering. The p-value of an exact Monte Carlo test based on the statistic (9.2) is $p = 0.14$, whereas the Normal approximation gives $p = 0.11$. We conclude that there is only very slight evidence of spatial clustering in these data, and that any clustering which may occur operates on a spatial scale of the order of several hundred metres.

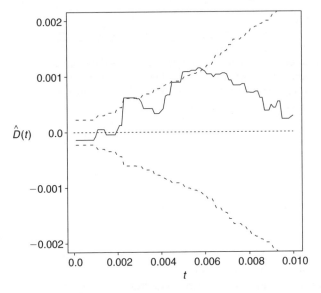

Figure 9.3. Second-order analysis of clustering for the North Humberside childhood leukaemia data: $\hat{D}(t)$ for observed data (solid curve); plus and minus two standard errors under random labelling of cases and controls. Unit of distance is 100 km.

9.2.2 Other tests of spatial clustering

In this context, there is no compelling reason to use the Diggle–Chetwynd statistic D. In fact, there is an extensive literature on tests of spatial clustering for epidemiological data, somewhat reminiscent of the burgeoning of tests of complete spatial randomness for ecological data 30 or more years ago, as reviewed in earlier chapters of this book. The idea of using case–control data, and the randomization distribution induced by the case–control design, to test for spatial clustering was introduced in Cuzick and Edwards (1990). Alexander and Boyle (1996) report on an empirical comparison amongst a number of different tests, based on their ability to detect clustering in a number of synthetic data-sets. Other recent contributions include Tango (1995, 2000), Anderson and Titterington (1997), Kulldorff (1997, 1999) and Williams *et al.* (2001).

Our preference for the Diggle–Chetwynd statistic stems from its roots in general point process methodology, rather than its performance in any specific power comparisons. In particular, the interpretation of $K(t)$ as a scaled expectation means that we can in turn interpret $D(t)$ as a scaled expected number of excess cases within distance t of a reference case, by comparison with a completely random pattern of disease incidence in the underlying population. Hence, at least in principle, it is possible to use $\hat{D}(t)$ not only to test the null hypothesis of no spatial clustering, but also to estimate the size and spatial scale of clustering if present. On the other hand, an implicit limitation of $\hat{D}(t)$ is that it is intended only to estimate general tendencies to clustering on spatial scales which are small relative to the dimensions of the study region. It is not designed to detect specific clusters, which might point to spatially localized risk factors, nor to investigate broad spatial trends in disease risk. Put in more formal terms, for a test of spatial clustering as here defined the null hypothesis under test is that disease risk is spatially constant *and* cases occur independently, whereas the implicit alternative is that risk remains constant, but cases are dependent.

Methods for detecting specific clusters of disease are sometimes called *focused tests*, to distinguish them from tests of clustering as described above. A good example, with a carefully argued rationale for their use in practice, is Besag and Newell (1991). In effect, these methods operate by testing whether particular concentrations of cases are statistically significant, with appropriate modifications to allow for the implicit multiple testing.

9.3 Spatial variation in risk

By *spatial variation in risk* we mean that the case and control intensity functions are not proportional. Specifically, let $r(x)$ denote the probability that a person at location x will be a case. Then, adopting the usual convention that controls must be non-cases, the respective intensity functions of cases and controls are

$$\lambda_1(x) = r(x)\lambda(x) \tag{9.3}$$

and

$$\lambda_2(x) = c\{1 - r(x)\}\lambda(x), \tag{9.4}$$

where $\lambda(x)$ is the intensity of the underlying population and c is a constant determined by the study design. It follows that $\lambda_1(x)$ and $\lambda_2(x)$ are proportional if and only if $r(x)$ is constant. The function $r(x)$ is called the *risk surface*.

In contrast to spatial clustering, spatial variation in risk *is* a description of the study region, under the implicit assumption that cases of disease occur independently of one another. As we have seen in earlier chapters, it can be difficult or even impossible to sustain an empirical distinction between a process of dependent events in a homogeneous environment and one of independent events in a heterogeneous environment. To emphasize this in the present context, the null hypothesis of no spatial variation in risk, $r(x) = r$, is equivalent to random labelling of cases and controls, which is also the hypothesis of no spatial clustering. Thus, spatial clustering and spatial variation in risk represent different alternatives to the same null hypothesis.

Conditional on the intensity surface $\lambda_1(x)$, and under the assumption that cases occur independently, the case map is a realization of an inhomogeneous Poisson process. Controls occur independently by design. It follows that, conditional on the intensity surface $\lambda_2(x)$, the control map is a realization of a second, independent Poisson process. Also, it follows from (9.3) and (9.4) that

$$\lambda_1(x)/\lambda_2(x) = c^{-1}r(x)/\{1 - r(x)\}. \tag{9.5}$$

This shows that, up to a multiplicative constant, disease odds $r(x)/\{1-r(x)\}$, and hence the risk surface $r(x)$, can be estimated non-parametrically via non-parametric estimates of the two intensity functions $\lambda_j(x)$. Specifically, we can estimate the risk surface by substituting into (9.5) kernel estimates of the $\lambda_j(x)$ as discussed in Section 8.2.

In order to choose values of h for the kernel estimates of the $\lambda_j(x)$, we could use the method described in Section 8.2. However, in the non-parametric setting, there is no reason to suppose that optimal values of h for separate estimation of the two functions $\lambda_j(x)$ will be optimal for their ratio. Kelsall and Diggle (1995a) show that

134 Statistical analysis of spatial point patterns

the asymptotically optimal estimator with respect to mean square error is achieved by using equal values of h in the numerator and denominator, irrespective of the numbers of cases and controls. Kelsall and Diggle (1995b) describe an application to data on cancer.

A second method of estimating the risk surface non-parametrically, due to Kelsall and Diggle (1998) is motivated by the following observation. Consider two independent Poisson processes with respective intensities $\lambda_1(x)$ and $\lambda_2(x)$. Then the superposition of the two is also a Poisson process, with intensity $\lambda_1(x) + \lambda_2(x)$. In this superposition, define a binary random variable Y_i to take the value 1 or 0 according to whether the ith event in the superposition is an event of the first or the second component process. Then, conditional on the superposition, the labels Y_i are mutually independent with

$$P(Y_i = 1) = \lambda_1(x_i)/\{\lambda_1(x_i) + \lambda_2(x_i)\}. \tag{9.6}$$

If we now substitute from (9.3) and (9.4) into the right-hand side of (9.6), we obtain

$$\log\{P(Y_i = 1)/P(Y_i = 0)\} = -\log c + \log[r(x_i)/\{1 - r(x_i)\}]. \tag{9.7}$$

It follows from (9.7) that we can estimate the log-odds of disease, up to an additive constant, by using a non-parametric logistic regression model for the binary responses Y_i. This approach has the important advantage over the kernel density ratio estimator that it is easily extended to incorporate covariate information attached to individual cases and controls. Specifically, if we define the log-odds function $\ell(x) = \log[r(x)/\{1 - r(x)\}]$ and let z_i denote a covariate vector for the ith individual (case or control), then a semi-parametric model to identify residual spatial variation after adjusting for covariate effects is

$$\log\{P(Y_i = 1)/P(Y_i = 0)\} = \alpha + z_i'\beta + \ell(x_i). \tag{9.8}$$

Note in particular that the z_i could include spatial effects, such as a measure of social deprivation, or non-spatial effects such as the age or sex of the ith individual.

If the function $\ell(x)$ in (9.8) were to be specified parametrically, a natural approach to parameter estimation would be to maximize the log-likelihood,

$$L = \sum y_i \log p_i + \sum (1 - y_i) \log(1 - p_i), \tag{9.9}$$

where $p_i = P(Y_i = 1)$ as specified by (9.8). In the semi-parametric setting an alternative method is to maximize a cross-validated version of the log-likelihood. This takes the same form as (9.9), except that each p_i is estimated from all data *except* the ith event. By choosing the kernel bandwidth parameter h to maximize the cross-validated form of the log-likelihood, we avoid the degenerate solution, corresponding formally to $h = 0$, in which p_i is estimated as 1 or 0 according to whether the ith event is a case or control, respectively.

9.4 Point source models

The question of spatial variation in risk arises very directly when it is suspected that adverse effects on health are caused by a specific source of environmental pollution. A much-studied, and controversial, example in the UK has been the investigation of unusually high incidences of childhood cancer near nuclear installations. See, for example, Cook-Mozaffari et al. (1989) and Gardner (1989).

In this more structured setting, it is reasonable to contemplate parametric modelling of the risk surface in relation to the postulated source. This leads to a general model in which controls and cases form independent Poisson processes with respective intensities $\lambda_2(x)$ and $\lambda_1(x) = \phi \lambda_2(x) \rho(x)$, where $\lambda_2(x)$ is of unspecified form, $\rho(x)$ is given by a parametric model and ϕ is a nuisance parameter which relates to the relative numbers of cases and controls, the latter being under the control of the investigator. Using the same argument as in Section 9.3 above, by considering case–control labels conditional on locations we can convert the Poisson process model to a binary regression model with spatially dependent probabilities

$$p(x) = \lambda_1(x)/\{\lambda_1(x) + \lambda_2(x)\} = \phi\rho(x)/\{1 + \phi\rho(x)\}, \quad (9.10)$$

thereby eliminating the nuisance function $\lambda_2(x)$.

We first consider models which depend only on distance from a point source. Hence, the risk at a location x is proportional to some function $\rho(\|x - x_0\|)$, where x_0 is the location of the source and $\|\cdot\|$ denotes distance.

The simplest possible such model postulates an elevation in risk within some critical distance δ say, hence

$$\rho(u) = \begin{cases} 1 + \alpha : u \leq \delta, \\ 1 : u > \delta. \end{cases}$$

In practice, this model is often used with a subjectively chosen value for δ (Elliott et al., 1992). The resulting analysis is extremely simple. In this setting, case–control locations can be reduced to a 2×2 contingency table of events classified by their case–control designations and their distance from the source being greater or less than δ. The test for elevated risk within the selected distance threshold is then a standard comparison of two binomial proportions, and the corresponding empirical proportions of cases, p_1 and p_2 say, from events below and above the distance threshold, estimate $1/\{1 + \phi(1 + \alpha)\}$ and $\phi(1 + \alpha)/\{1 + \phi(1 + \alpha)\}$, respectively.

Lawson (1989), Diggle (1990) and Diggle and Rowlingson (1994) used an isotropic Gaussian model,

$$\rho(u) = 1 + \alpha \exp\{-(u/\delta)^2\}. \quad (9.11)$$

As in the previous model, the parameter α measures the elevation in risk at the source, whereas δ measures the rate at which risk decays smoothly with increasing distance towards a background level represented by $\rho = 1$. Whilst there is no particular theoretical justification for assuming the Gaussian shape, a smoothly decaying risk function will be qualitatively sensible in many applications. Also, (9.11) meets the dual requirement of a finite value for $\rho(0)$ and a positive value for $\rho(u)$ as $u \to \infty$. These requirements, together with the fact that a well-designed study will seek to establish the range over which any elevation in risk operates, rule out the use of standard generalized linear models.

Ideally, the form of model should be suggested by the practical context, for example to correspond to the behaviour of a plume of dispersing pollutant. This analogy immediately raises the possibility that the pattern of elevation in risk may have a directional component. As a simple example of how a directional effect might be incorporated, Figure 9.4 shows examples of a directional model with

$$\rho(u, \theta) = 1 + \alpha \exp(-[u \exp\{\kappa \cos(\theta - \phi)\}/\beta]^2). \quad (9.12)$$

136 *Statistical analysis of spatial point patterns*

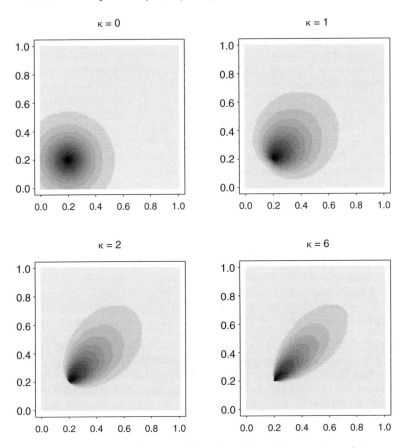

Figure 9.4. Examples of a directional model for elevation in risk around a point source, with different values of the parameter κ in (9.12).

In (9.12), α represents the elevation in risk at the source, β the rate of decay of risk with distance from the source, ϕ the principal direction of the plume and κ the extent of directional concentration of the plume, hence each of the parameters has a tangible interpretation. Lawson (1993) models directional effects by including terms $\cos(\theta - \phi)$ and $u \cos(\theta - \phi)$ in a log-linear formulation for $\rho(\cdot)$.

In practice, point source models are rarely derived from theoretical arguments. More often, they are used simply as parsimonious, descriptive models. As in the non-parametric case, it is important to include adjustments for known available risk factors in order to avoid the detection of spurious spatial effects. For example, pollution sources are often sited in areas with generally higher than average social deprivation, which is known to be a risk factor for many diseases.

All of the specific point source models described above correspond formally to non-linear binary regression models for the case–control labels, and the properties of maximum likelihood estimation for such models, based on the log-likelihood function (9.9), may well show irregular behaviour. This is discussed, for example, in Diggle *et al.* (1997).

Table 9.1. Deviances (minus twice maximized log-likelihoods) for various sub-models fitted to the North Derbyshire childhood asthma data

Risk factors included	Deviance	Number of parameters
None	1165.9	2
Coking works	1160.7	4
Coking works, main roads	1160.6	6
Coking works, smoking	1159.4	5
Coking works, hay fever	1127.6	5
Hay fever only	1132.5	3

9.4.1 Childhood asthma in North Derbyshire, England

Diggle and Rowlingson (1994) fit the isotropic Gaussian model to data from a case–control study of asthmatic symptoms in elementary schools in North Derbyshire, England. The study population consisted of all children attending one of 10 schools in the area. Schools were stratified according to whether the headteacher had previously reported concern about the apparently high level of asthmatic symptoms in the school. Four potential sources were considered. Here we look only at two: a coking works, and the main road network. In the latter case, we used the distance between each child's residential location x and the nearest point on the road network as the distance measure in the model. Additional binary covariates for each child in the study indicated whether the household included at least one cigarette smoker, and whether the child suffered from hay fever. The overall risk was modelled multiplicatively, with separate terms for each of the two sources, and log-linear covariate adjustments for smoking, hay fever and the prior stratification of the schools into two groups.

Likelihood ratio comparisons within this overall modelling framework are summarized in Table 9.1. The conclusions from Table 9.1 are that hay fever is the biggest single risk factor, and is overwhelmingly significant, and that proximity to the coking works shows a marginally significant increase in risk, with or without prior adjustment for hay fever. For example, the comparison between the last two lines of the table gives a chi-squared value of 4.9 on 2 degrees of freedom to test the association with the coke works after adjusting for hay fever. There is no evidence of significant association with main roads, or with cigarette smoking.

9.4.2 Cancers in North Liverpool

We now present the results of an investigation which used both parametric and non-parametric approaches to the estimation of spatial variation in risk. The investigation concerned the spatial distribution of cancer cases in an area of North Liverpool, UK, in which specific concerns had been expressed about possible elevation in risk near the site of a now disused hospital incinerator. The results presented below are extracted from Ardern (2001).

The study used an unmatched case–control design. The case locations consisted of the residential post-codes of all known cases of cancer diagnosed between 1974 and 1988. Adult cancers were classified into seven types, as shown in Table 9.2.

Table 9.2. Numbers of North Liverpool cancer cases available for analysis

Type	Number
Colorectal	1162
Lung	2345
Liver	70
Larynx and nasopharynx	126
Leukaemia and lymphoma	365
Soft tissue sarcoma	45
Other cancers	5828
Total	9941

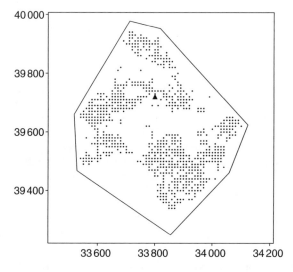

Figure 9.5. Study region and control locations for North Liverpool cancer study. The solid triangle shows the location of the now disused hospital incinerator. Axis labels are grid reference northings and eastings.

A random sample of 10 000 control locations was drawn from a database of general practitioner registrations within the study area, as shown in Figure 9.5. Also shown in Figure 9.5 is the location of the former incinerator. Covariate information attached to each case or control consisted of the individual's age and sex, and the Townsend index of social deprivation for the census enumeration district containing the individual's residential location (Townsend *et al.*, 1988).

The initial analysis consisted of fitting the isotropic model (9.11), based on distance from the former incinerator and including log-linear adjustments for age, sex and the Townsend index. For all types of cancer, after adjustment for covariate effects the association with distance from the incinerator was non-significant. Table 9.3 shows the estimated covariate adjustments and their significance. As expected, the effect of age is highly significant and positive for all adult cancer types considered. The effect of sex is highly significant for colorectal, lung and larynx/nasopharynx cancers, with risk higher

Table 9.3. Parameter estimates of regression effects associated with sex, age and social deprivation, and p-values for associated likelihood ratio tests of significance

Cancer type	Parameter estimate			p-value		
	age	sex	depriv	age	sex	depriv
Colorectal	0.076	−0.31	0.033	<0.001	<0.001	<0.001
Lung	0.077	−0.97	0.086	<0.001	<0.001	<0.001
Liver	0.062	−0.56	0.071	<0.001	0.02	0.06
Larynx/nasopharynx	0.059	−1.34	0.125	<0.001	<0.001	<0.001
Leukaemia/lymphoma	0.048	−0.30	0.043	<0.001	0.005	0.01
Soft tissue sarcoma	0.045	−0.32	−0.048	<0.001	0.29	0.28
All adult cancers	0.075	−0.14	0.036	<0.001	<0.001	<0.001

for men than for women. Sex is less significant for liver and for leukaemias/lymphomas and non-significant for soft tissue sarcomas, although this may be a reflection of the smaller sample sizes available for the less common cancer types. Social deprivation as measured by the Townsend index is highly significant for colorectal, lung and larynx/nasopharynx cancers, and less significant or non-significant for the remaining, less common types. This may again be a reflection of the smaller sample sizes available, rather than absence of a genuine effect. In all cases, the association with distance from the incinerator is non-significant.

The conclusion from the initial analysis is therefore that there is no significant evidence of association between cancer risk and the location of the former incinerator. To investigate the possibility of unexplained spatial variation in risk *not* associated with the incinerator, we used the semi-parametric model (9.8) as described in Section 9.3, again adjusting for age, sex and social deprivation. The kernel smoothing term used a quartic kernel with a subjectively chosen bandwidth $h = 0.5$ km. The method was used only on the more common cancer types, as the non-parametric smoothing requires a large sample size to be effective. Figures 9.6–9.8 show the resulting estimates of residual spatial variation in risk. In each case, the scale is logarithmic to base 2, hence each unit increase in the grey-scale corresponds to a doubling of estimated risk. The solid and dashed contours identify regions within which the local risk is pointwise significantly higher or lower, respectively, than the average for the whole study area, at the 5% level. Common to all three types is an area of apparently elevated risk close to the north-eastern boundary of the study area. The p-values for an overall test of departure from constant residual risk are 0.05, 0.01 and 0.67 for colorectal, lung and leukaemia/lymphoma, respectively. This suggests that, at least for colorectal and lung cancers, the elevated risk close to the north-eastern boundary is genuinely significant, rather than an artefact of implicit multiple testing.

9.5 Stratification and matching

9.5.1 Stratified case–control designs

All of the methods described above are easily adapted to stratified case–control studies. Provided the number of events within each stratum is sufficiently large, the analysis can be carried out separately within each stratum and the results pooled as and when

140 *Statistical analysis of spatial point patterns*

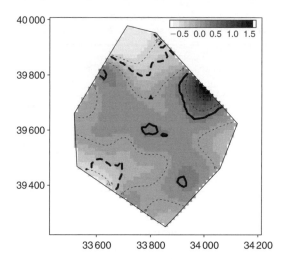

Figure 9.6. Estimated residual spatial variation in risk for colorectal cancers in the North Liverpool study. The risk scale is logarithmic to base 2. Solid and dashed contours identify regions within which risk is pointwise 5% significantly higher or lower, respectively, than the average for the whole study area.

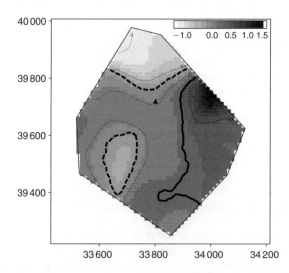

Figure 9.7. Estimated residual spatial variation in risk for lung cancers in the North Liverpool study. The risk scale is logarithmic to base 2. Solid and dashed contours identify regions within which risk is pointwise 5% significantly higher or lower, respectively, than the average for the whole study area.

appropriate. The precise form of pooling will depend on what supplementary assumptions are considered to be reasonable. We illustrate this for the specific case in which there are two strata, for example one for each sex.

We first consider how to modify a test for spatial clustering when cases and controls can each be divided into two strata. Compute test statistics D_1 and D_2 within each

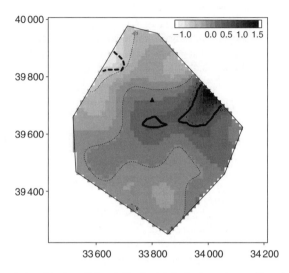

Figure 9.8. Estimated residual spatial variation in risk for leukaemias and lymphomas in the North Liverpool study. The risk scale is logarithmic to base 2. Solid and dashed contours identify regions within which risk is pointwise 5% significantly higher or lower, respectively, than the average for the whole study area.

stratum, as described in Section 9.2. If v_j denotes the null variance of D_j according to the Diggle–Chetwynd formula, then a suitable combined test statistic is given by $D = v_1^{-0.5} D_1 + v_2^{-0.5} D_2$. Under the reasonable assumption that the labelling processes operating in the two strata are independent, the null expectation and variance of D are 0 and 2, respectively. An approximate test follows by assuming a Normal sampling distribution for D, whereas an exact, Monte Carlo test is available by jointly relabelling cases and controls randomly within each stratum.

We now consider non-parametric estimation of a spatially varying risk surface when there are two strata. In this case, we use the generalized additive model formulation (9.8). The simplest way to incorporate strata into the analysis is then as a two-level factor to be added to the model as a main effect. If necessary, the stratum factor could then be allowed to interact with other terms in the model.

For the parametric modelling of elevated risk near a point source, the same basic strategy applies. We introduce the stratum label as a two-level factor, to be added to the regression model either as a main effect, or as an interaction with other terms.

These methods of dealing with data in two strata extend in the obvious way to $k > 2$ strata. However, in practice this is only a useful strategy if the number of strata is small and the numbers of events within strata are large.

9.5.2 Individually matched case–control designs

When strata are small, a different approach is needed. We consider here the setting of individually matched data, whereby each case is associated with a set of k controls matched to the corresponding case by the values of one or more identifiable factors.

To investigate spatial clustering in this setting, Chetwynd et al. (2001) evaluate the null expectation and covariance structure of $\hat{D}(t) = \hat{K}_{11}(t) - \hat{K}_{22}(t)$ for an individually matched case–control design. They show that when $k = 1$, the null expectation of $D(t)$ is still zero, whereas when $k > 1$ it is non-zero, perhaps substantially so. This suggests that we should modify the test statistic (9.2), for example to

$$D' = \int_0^{t_0} v(t)^{-0.5} \{\hat{D}(t) - \mu(t)\} dt,$$

where $\mu(t)$ denotes the null expectation of $D(t)$, and $v(t)$ now denotes the variance calculated from the randomization distribution appropriate to the individually matched design.

An intuitive explanation of the non-zero null expectation in the case $k > 1$ is that the matching variables may themselves be spatially non-neutral. For example, suppose that marginally the population, and hence the cases under the null hypothesis of no spatial clustering, are distributed completely at random, but that matched controls are likely to be spatially close to the corresponding case. Then the cases would generate an estimate $\hat{K}_{11}(t) \approx \pi t^2$, but when $k > 1$ the controls would tend to fall in clumps of size k, leading to $\hat{K}_{22}(t) > \pi t^2$. This kind of effect can easily arise in practice because administrative, demographic or socioeconomic factors, which are often used as matching variables, tend to be spatially non-neutral. A corollary is that individual matching can easily induce spurious spatial effects if the analysis fails to make allowance for the matching in the study design.

For non-parametric or parametric modelling of spatial variation in risk using the binary regression formulation, individual matching requires the basic form of the likelihood function introduced in Section 9.3 to be modified. Let $p(x)$ denote the probability that a person at location x is a case, and x_{ij} the location of the jth member of the ith matched case–control set with $i = 1$ identifying the case and $i = 2, \ldots, k+1$ its matched controls. Then, the matched design is equivalent to a constraint that amongst the $k+1$ members of any matched set there is exactly one case. The probability that the case is the member at location x_{i1} is therefore given by

$$p_j = p(x_{i1}) \Big/ \sum_{i=1}^{k+1} p(x_{ij}).$$

The corresponding log-likelihood for n matched sets is given by

$$L^* = \sum_{j=1}^{n} \log p_j, \qquad (9.13)$$

which is to be compared with the corresponding expression (9.9) for a randomized case–control design.

Diggle, Morris and Wakefield (2000) discuss inference based on the log-likelihood (9.13) in the specific context of point source models. Jarner et al. (2002) discuss non-parametric estimation of the risk surface. As in the case of spatial clustering, when matching variables are spatially non-neutral they introduce an ambiguity into precisely what is being estimated as a spatial effect. For this reason, when spatial variation is of particular interest, we would recommend dealing with measurable risk factors by regression adjustments where possible, rather than by individual matching at the design stage. Of course, it remains true that spatial effects will usually only be of scientific interest if they persist after adjustment for all known risk factors, whether or not these are themselves spatially structured.

9.5.3 Is stratification or matching helpful?

In general, epidemiologists are divided on the merits of stratification and/or matching over the completely randomized design, for the good reason that there are clear advantages and disadvantages to the more complex designs and the balance between the different considerations will inevitably change in different practical settings. See, for example, Woodward (1999, pp. 266–8).

When spatial variation is a major scientific focus, the author's opinion is that fine stratification or individual matching are undesirable, because they severely complicate the interpretation of the estimated spatial effect. Specifically, consider the problem of estimating residual spatial variation in risk in a stratified design. As noted above, the analysis proceeds in the first instance by adding stratum effects to the generalized additive model (9.8). If we now let Y_{ij} take the value 1 if the jth event in the ith stratum is a case, and the value 0 if it is a control, and write $p_{ij} = P(Y_{ij} = 1)$, then the model for the data is that the Y_{ij} are mutually independent with

$$\log\{p_{ij}/(1 - p_{ij})\} = \alpha_i + z'_{ij}\beta + \ell(x_{ij}) \tag{9.14}$$

where x_{ij} and z_{ij} respectively denote the location and covariate vector associated with Y_{ij}. In the extreme case of individual matching, or more generally when there are many strata, the standard analysis uses the log-likelihood (9.13) to estimate β and $\ell(\cdot)$ whilst eliminating the nuisance parameters α_i. However, and especially when $\ell(\cdot)$ is specified non-parametrically, the interpretation of the resulting estimate of the spatial surface $\ell(x)$ is now problematic. Suppose, for example, that the events within a particular stratum are concentrated within a small sub-region of the whole study region. Then the presence of the α_i parameter in (9.14), coupled with its elimination from the stratified log-likelihood (9.13), means in effect that the behaviour of the spatial surface $\ell(x)$ in that sub-region is only identifiable up to an arbitrary constant. More generally, one of the advantages claimed for stratified or matched designs is to eliminate the effects of the matching variables on the presumption that these are not of scientific interest; but if the matching variables are not spatially neutral, then they are partially confounded with the spatial effect, which for the purposes of the present discussion *is* of scientific interest.

9.6 Disentangling heterogeneity and clustering

An issue which arises quite generally in the analysis of spatial point process data, but which is particularly obvious in epidemiological applications, is the difficulty of separating variation in intensity from clustering of events. We have shown how the case–control paradigm can resolve the difficulty with respect to testing a null hypothesis which specifies no variation in intensity *and* no clustering, but it leaves ambiguous the interpretation of a significant test result.

In other branches of statistics which deal with dependent data, for example in the analysis of real-valued spatial data, the usual pragmatic strategy is to partition the data into the sum of a spatially varying mean value function and random variation about the mean, hence $Y(x) = \mu(x) + Z(x)$, where $Y(\cdot)$ is the observed process, $\mu(x) = E[Y(x)]$ and $Z(\cdot)$ is a zero-mean residual process (see, for example, Chiles and Delfiner, 1999). The analogous modelling assumption for point process data is to allow a non-constant intensity $\lambda(x)$ but to assume that the higher-order random variation is, in some sense, stationary. One way to formalize this, as discussed in Section 4.2, is to assume that the process is *reweighted second-order stationary*, meaning that $\lambda_2(x, y)/\{\lambda(x)\lambda(y)\} = \rho(t)$, where t is the distance between x and y. For processes of this kind, the definition of the K-function extends naturally to

$$K_I(t) = 2\pi \int_0^t \rho(x) x \, dx$$

although, as discussed in Section 4.6.2, estimation of $K_I(t)$ from a single realization is problematic.

In the case–control setting, there is a much clearer rationale for separate estimation of a spatially varying $\lambda(x)$ and stationary second-order properties. By construction, a random sample of controls constitutes a realization of an inhomogeneous Poisson process, albeit one with a possibly very complicated intensity function, and the controls can be used to estimate the surface $\lambda(x)$. Given an estimate $\hat{\lambda}(x)$, we can then use the case data to estimate $\rho(t)$ or, equivalently, $K_I(t)$, incorporating the control-based estimate $\hat{\lambda}(x)$. This idea is currently being developed by Susan Gooding in a Lancaster University PhD; her preliminary results indicate, for example, that a test for spatial clustering based on the empirical function $\hat{K}_I(t) - \pi t^2$ is more powerful than the Diggle–Chetwynd approach of comparing estimated homogeneous K-functions for cases and controls. These results will be reported formally in due course.

References

Alexander, F.E. and Boyle, P. (1996). *Methods for Investigating Localized Clustering of Disease.* Lyon: International Agency for Research on Cancer.

Anderson, N.H. and Titterington, D.M. (1997). Some methods for investigating spatial clustering, with epidemiological applications. *Journal of the Royal Statistical Society*, A **160**, 87–105.

Ardern, K. (2001). *Report on the Possible Increase in Cancer Cases in North Liverpool and Potential Links to the Site of the Former Incinerator at Fazakerley Hospital.* Liverpool: Liverpool Health Authority.

Baddeley, A.J. (1999). Spatial sampling and censoring. In *Stochastic Geometry: Likelihood and Computation*, ed. O.E. Barndorff-Nielsen, W.S. Kendall and M.N.M. Van Lieshout, 37–78. London: Chapman & Hall.

Baddeley, A.J. and Møller, J. (1989). Nearest-neighbour Markov point processes and random sets. *International Statistical Review*, **57**, 89–121.

Baddeley, A.J., Møller, J. and Waagepetersen, R. (2000). Non- and semi-parametric estimation of interaction in inhomogeneous point patterns. *Statistica Neerlandica*, **54**, 329–50.

Baddeley, A.J., Moyeed, R.A., Howard, C.V. and Boyde, A. (1993). Analysis of a three-dimensional point pattern with replication. *Applied Statistics*, **42**, 641–68.

Baddeley, A.J. and Silverman, B.S. (1984). A cautionary example on the use of second-order methods for analyzing point patterns. *Biometrics*, **40**, 1089–93.

Baddeley, A. and Turner, R. (2000). Practical maximum pseudolikelihood for spatial point patterns (with discussion). *Australian and New Zealand Journal of Statistics*, **42**, 283–322.

Baddeley, A.J. and Van Lieshout, M.N.M. (1995). Area-interaction point processes. *Annals of the Institute of Statistical Mathematics*, **47**, 601–19.

Bailey, T.C. and Gatrell, A.G. (1995). *Interactive Spatial Data Analysis.* Harlow: Longman.

Barnard, G.A. (1963). Contribution to the discussion of Professor Bartlett's paper. *Journal of the Royal Statistical Society*, B **25**, 294.

Bartlett, M.S. (1937). Properties of sufficiency and statistical tests. *Proceedings of the Royal Society*, A **160**, 268–82.

Bartlett, M.S. (1964). Spectral analysis of two-dimensional point processes. *Biometrika*, **51**, 299–311.

Bartlett, M.S. (1971). Two-dimensional nearest neighbour systems and their ecological applications. In *Statistical Ecology*, Vol. 1, ed. G.P. Patil, E.C. Pielou and W.E. Waters, 179–84. University Park: Pennsylvania State University Press.

Bartlett, M.S. (1975). *The Statistical Analysis of Spatial Pattern.* London: Chapman & Hall.

Berman, M. and Diggle, P. (1989). Estimating weighted integrals of the second-order intensity of a spatial point process. *Journal of the Royal Statistical Society*, B **51**, 81–92.

Berman, M. and Turner, T.R. (1992). Approximating point process likelihoods with GLIM. *Applied Statistics*, **41**, 31–8.

Bernal, J.D. (1960). Geometry of the structure of monatomic liquids. *Nature*, **185**, 68–70.

References

Besag, J. (1974). Spatial interaction and the statistical analysis of lattice systems (with discussion). *Journal of the Royal Statistical Society*, B **34**, 192–236.

Besag, J. (1975). Statistical analysis of non-lattice data. *The Statistician*, **24**, 179–95.

Besag, J. (1977). Contribution to the discussion of Dr Ripley's paper. *Journal of the Royal Statistical Society*, B **39**, 193–5.

Besag, J. (1978). Some methods of statistical analysis for spatial data. *Bulletin of the International Statistical Institute*, **47**, 77–92.

Besag, J. and Diggle, P.J. (1977). Simple Monte Carlo tests for spatial pattern. *Applied Statistics*, **26**, 327–33.

Besag, J. and Gleaves, J.T. (1973). On the detection of spatial pattern in plant communities. *Bulletin of the International Statistical Institute*, **45**(1), 153–8.

Besag, J., Milne, R. and Zachary, S. (1982). Point process limits of lattice processes. *Journal of Applied Probability*, **19**, 210–16.

Besag, J. and Newell, J. (1991). The detection of clusters of rare diseases. *Journal of the Royal Statistical Society*, A **154**, 143–55.

Breslow, N.E. and Day, N.E. (1980). *Statistical Methods in Cancer Research, Volume 1: The Analysis of Case–Control Studies*. Lyon: International Agency for Research on Cancer.

Brown, D. (1975). A test of randomness of nest spacing. *Wildfowl*, **26**, 102–3.

Brown, D. and Rothery, P. (1978). Randomness and local regularity of points in a plane. *Biometrika*, **65**, 115–22.

Brown, S. and Holgate, P. (1974). The thinned plantation. *Biometrika*, **61**, 253–62.

Brown, T. (1979). Position dependent and stochastic thinning of point processes. *Stochastic Processes and Their Applications*, **9**, 189–93.

Byth, K. (1982). On robust distance-based intensity estimators. *Biometrics*, **38**, 127–35.

Byth, K. and Ripley, B. D. (1980). On sampling spatial patterns by distance methods. *Biometrics*, **36**, 279–84.

Catana, A.J. (1963). The wandering quarter method of estimating population density. *Ecology*, **44**, 349–60.

Chetwynd, A.G. and Diggle, P.J. (1998). On estimating the reduced second moment measure of a stationary spatial point process. *Australian and New Zealand Journal of Statistics*, **40**, 11–15.

Chetwynd, A.G., Diggle, P.J., Marshall, A. and Parslow, R. (2001). Investigation of spatial clustering from individually matched case–control studies. *Biostatistics*, **2**, 277–93.

Chiles, J.-P. and Delfiner, P. (1999). *Geostatistics*. New York: Wiley.

Clark, P.J. and Evans, F.C. (1954). Distance to nearest neighbour as a measure of spatial relationships in populations. *Ecology*, **35**, 23–30.

Cliff, A.D. and Ord, J.K. (1981). *Spatial Processes: Models and Applications*. London: Pion.

Cook-Mozaffari, P., Darby, S., Doll, R., Forman, D., Hermon, C. and Pike, M.C. (1989). Geographical variation in mortality from leukaemia and other cancers in England and Wales in relation to proximity to nuclear installations, 1969–78. *British Journal of Cancer*, **59**, 476–85.

Cormack, R.M. (1977). The invariance of Cox and Lewis' statistic for the analysis of spatial patterns. *Biometrika*, **64**, 143–4.

Cormack, R.M. (1979). Spatial aspects of competition between individuals. In *Spatial and Temporal Analysis in Ecology*, ed. R.M. Cormack and J.K. Ord, 152–211. Fairland, MD: International Co-operative Publishing House.

Cottam, G. and Curtis, J. T. (1949). A method for making rapid surveys of woodlands, by means of pairs of randomly selected trees. *Ecology*, **30**, 101–4.

Cox, D.R. (1955). Some statistical methods related with series of events (with discussion). *Journal of the Royal Statistical Society*, B **17**, 129–64.

Cox, D.R. (1972). The statistical analysis of dependencies in point processes. In *Stochastic Point Processes*, ed. P.A.W. Lewis, 55–66. New York: Wiley.

Cox, D.R. (1977). The role of significance tests. *Scandinavian Journal of Statistics*, **4**, 49–70.

Cox, D.R. and Lewis, P.A.W. (1966). *The Statistical Analysis of Series of Events*. London: Methuen.
Cox, D.R. and Lewis, P.A.W. (1972). Multivariate point processes. In *Proceedings of the Sixth Berkeley Symposium on Mathematical Statistics and Probability*, ed. L. Le Cam, J. Neyman and E.L. Scott, Vol. 3, 401–448. Berkeley: University of California Press.
Cox, T.F. (1976). The robust estimation of the density of a forest stand using a new conditioned distance method. *Biometrika*, **63**, 493–500.
Cox, T.F. and Lewis, T. (1976). A conditioned distance ratio method for analysing spatial patterns. *Biometrika*, **63**, 483–92.
Cressie, N.A.C. (1991). *Statistics for Spatial Data*. New York: Wiley.
Crick, F.H.C. and Lawrence, P.A. (1975). Compartments and polychones in insect development. *Science*, **189**, 340–7.
Cuzick, J. and Edwards, R. (1990). Spatial clustering for inhomogeneous populations (with discussion). *Journal of the Royal Statistical Society*, B **52**, 73–104.
Daley, D.J. and Vere-Jones, D. (1972). A summary of the theory of point processes. In *Stochastic Point Processes*, ed. P.A.W. Lewis, 299–383. New York: Wiley.
Diggle, P.J. (1975). Robust density estimation using distance methods. *Biometrika*, **62**, 39–48.
Diggle, P.J. (1977a). A note on robust density estimation for spatial point patterns. *Biometrika*, **64**, 91–5.
Diggle, P.J. (1977b). The detection of random heterogeneity in plant populations. *Biometrics*, **33**, 390–4.
Diggle, P.J. (1978). On parameter estimation for spatial point processes. *Journal of the Royal Statistical Society*, B **40**, 178–81.
Diggle, P.J. (1979a). On parameter estimation and goodness-of-fit testing for spatial point patterns. *Biometrics*, **35**, 87–101.
Diggle, P.J. (1985a). Displaced amacrine cells in the retina of a rabbit: analysis of a bivariate spatial point pattern. *Journal of Neuroscience Methods*, **18**, 115–25.
Diggle, P.J. (1985b). A kernel method for smoothing point process data. *Applied Statistics*, **34**, 138–47.
Diggle, P.J. (1990). A point process modelling approach to raised incidence of a rare phenomenon in the vicinity of a prespecified point. *Journal of the Royal Statistical Society*, A **153**, 349–62.
Diggle, P., Besag, J. and Gleaves, J.T. (1976). Statistical analysis of spatial point patterns by means of distance methods. *Biometrics*, **32**, 659–67.
Diggle, P.J. and Chetwynd, A.G. (1991). Second-order analysis of spatial clustering for inhomogeneous populations. *Biometrics*, **47**, 1155–63.
Diggle, P.J. and Cox, T.F. (1981). On sparse sampling methods and tests of independence for multivariate spatial point patterns. *Bulletin of the International Statistical Institute*, **49**.
Diggle, P., Elliott, P., Morris, S. and Shaddick, G. (1997). Regression modelling of disease risk in relation to point sources. *Journal of the Royal Statistical Society*, A **160**, 491–505.
Diggle, P.J., Fiksel, T., Grabarnik, P., Ogata, Y., Stoyan, D. and Tanemura, M. (1994). On parameter estimation for pairwise interaction point processes. *International Statistical Review*, **62**, 99–117.
Diggle, P.J., Gates, D.J. and Stibbard, A. (1987). A non-parametric estimator for pairwise-interaction point processes. *Biometrika*, **74**, 763–70.
Diggle, P.J. and Gratton, R.J. (1984). Monte Carlo methods of inference for implicit statistical models (with discussion). *Journal of the Royal Statistical Society*, B **46**, 193–227.
Diggle, P.J., Lange, N. and Benes, F.M. (1991). Analysis of variance for replicated spatial point patterns in clinical neuroanatomy. *Journal of the American Statistical Association*, **86**, 618–25.
Diggle, P.J. and Matérn, B. (1981). On sampling designs for the estimation of point–event nearest neighbour distributions. *Scandinavian Journal of Statistics*, **7**, 80–4.

Diggle, P.J., Mateu, J. and Clough, H.E. (2000). A comparison between parametric and nonparametric approaches to the analysis of replicated spatial point patterns. *Advances in Applied Probability*, **32**, 331–43.

Diggle, P.J. and Milne, R.K. (1983a). Negative binomial quadrat counts and point processes. *Scandinavian Journal of Statistics*, **10**, 257–67.

Diggle, P.J. and Milne, R.K. (1983b). Bivariate Cox processes: some models for bivariate spatial point patterns. *Journal of the Royal Statistical Society*, B **45**, 11–21.

Diggle, P.J., Morris, S.E. and Wakefield, J.C. (2000). Point-source modelling using matched case–control data. *Biostatistics*, **1**, 89–105.

Diggle, P.J. and Rowlingson, B.S. (1994). A conditional approach to point process modelling of elevated risk. *Journal of the Royal Statistical Society*, A **157**, 433–40.

Donnelly, K. (1978). Simulations to determine the variance and edge-effect of total nearest neighbour distance. In *Simulation Methods in Archaeology*, ed. I. Hodder, 91–5. London: Cambridge University Press.

Douglas, J.B. (1979). *Analysis with Standard Contagious Distributions*. Fairland, MD: International Co-operative Publishing House.

Du Rietz, G.E. (1929). The fundamental units of vegetation. *Proceedings of the International Congress of Plant Science, Ithaca*, **1**, 623–7.

Eberhardt, L.L. (1967). Some developments in "distance sampling". *Biometrics*, **23**, 207–16.

Efron, B. and Tibshirani, R.J. (1993). *An Introduction to the Bootstrap*. London: Chapman & Hall.

Elliott, P., Beresford, J.A., Jolley, D.J., Pattenden, S.H. and Hills, M. (1992). Cancer of the larynx and lung near incinerators of waste solvents and oils in Britain. In *Geographical and Environmental Epidemiology: Methods for Small-Area Studies*, ed. P. Elliott, J. Cuzick, D. English and R. Stern, 359–67. Oxford: Oxford University Press.

Elliott, P., Wakefield, J.C., Best, N.G. and Briggs, D.J. (2000). *Spatial Epidemiology: Methods and Applications*. Oxford: Oxford University Press.

Evans, D.A. (1953). Experimental evidence concerning contagious distributions in ecology. *Biometrika*, **40**, 186–211.

Feller, W. (1968). *An Introduction to Probability Theory and its Applications*, Vol. 1, 3rd edn. New York: Wiley.

Fisher, R.A., Thornton, H.G. and Mackenzie, W. A. (1922). The accuracy of the plating method of estimating the density of bacterial populations, with particular reference to the use of Thornton's agar medium with soil samples. *Annals of Applied Botany*, **9**, 325–59.

Gardner, M.J. (1989). Review of reported incidences of childhood cancer rates in the vicinity of nuclear installations in the U.K. *Journal of the Royal Statistical Society*, A **152**, 307–25.

Gates, D.J. and Westcott, M. (1986). Clustering estimates in spatial point distributions with unstable potentials. *Annals of the Institute of Statistical Mathematics*, **38 A**, 55–67.

Gerrard, D.J. (1969). Competition quotient: a new measure of the competition affecting individual forest trees. Research Bulletin No. 20, Agricultural Experiment Station, Michigan State University.

Geyer, C.J. (1999). Likelihood inference for spatial point processes. In *Stochastic Geometry, Likelihood and Computation*, ed. O.E. Barndorff-Nielsen, W.S. Kendall and M.N.M. Van Lieshout, 79–140. London: Chapman & Hall.

Geyer, C.J. and Thompson, E.A. (1992). Constrained Monte Carlo maximum likelihood for dependent data (with discussion). *Journal of the Royal Statistical Society*, B **54**, 657–99.

Ghent, A.W. (1963). Studies of regeneration of forest stands devastated by spruce budworm. *Forest Science*, **9**, 295–310.

Gilks, W.R., Richardson, S. and Spiegelhalter, D.J. (1996). *Markov Chain Monte Carlo in Practice*. London: Chapman & Hall.

Gill, P.E. and Murray, W. (1972). Quasi-Newton methods for unconstrained optimization. *Journal of the Institute of Mathematics and its Applications*, **9**, 91–108.
Goodall, D.G. (1965). Plotless tests of inter-specific association. *Journal of Ecology*, **53**, 197–210.
Green, P.J. and Sibson, R. (1978). Computing Dirichlet tessellations in the plane. *Computer Journal*, **21**, 168–73.
Greenland, S. and Morgenstern, H. (1989). Ecological bias, confounding and effect modification. *International Journal of Epidemiology*, **18**, 269–74.
Greig-Smith, P. (1952). The use of random and contiguous quadrats in the study of the structure of plant communities. *Annals of Botany*, **16**, 293–316.
Greig-Smith, P. (1964). *Quantitative Plant Ecology*, 2nd edn. London: Butterworth.
Greig-Smith, P. (1979). Pattern in vegetation. *Journal of Ecology*, **67**, 755–79.
Harkness, R.D. and Isham, V. (1983). A bivariate spatial point pattern of ants' nests. *Applied Statistics*, **32**, 293–303.
Heikkinen, J. and Penttinen, A. (1999). Bayesian smoothing in the estimation of the pair potential function of Gibbs point processes. *Bernoulli*, **5**, 1119–36.
Hines, W.G.S. and O'Hara Hines, R.J. (1979). The Eberhardt index and the detection of non-randomness of spatial point distributions. *Biometrika*, **66**, 73–80.
Hodder, I. and Orton, C. (1976). *Spatial Analysis in Archaeology*. London: Cambridge University Press.
Högmander, H. and Särkkä, A. (1999). Multitype spatial point patterns with hierarchical interactions. *Biometrics*, **55**, 1051–8.
Holgate, P. (1964). The efficiency of nearest neighbour estimators. *Biometrics*, **20**, 647–9.
Holgate, P. (1965a). Tests of randomness based on distance methods. *Biometrika*, **52**, 345–53.
Holgate, P. (1965b). Some new tests of randomness. *Journal of Ecology*, **53**, 261–6.
Holgate, P. (1965c). The distance from a random point to the nearest point of a closely packed lattice. *Biometrika*, **52**, 261–3.
Holgate, P. (1972). The use of distance methods for the analysis of spatial distributions of points. In *Stochastic Point Processes*, ed. P.A.W. Lewis, 122–53. New York: Wiley.
Hope, A.C.A. (1968). A simplified Monte Carlo significance test procedure. *Journal of the Royal Statistical Society*, B **30**, 582–98.
Hopkins, B. (1954). A new method of determining the type of distribution of plant individuals. *Annals of Botany*, **18**, 213–26.
Hsuan, F. (1979). Generating uniform polygonal random pairs. *Applied Statistics*, **28**, 170–2.
Hughes, A. (1981). Cat retina and the sampling theorem: the relation of transient and sustained brisk-unit cut-off frequency to α and β-mode cell density. *Experimental Brain Research*, **42**, 196–202.
Hutchings, M.J. (1979). Standing crop and pattern in pure stands of *Mercurialis perennis* and *Rubus fruticosus* in mixed deciduous woodland. *Oikos*, **31**, 351–7.
Jarner, M.F., Diggle, P.J. and Chetwynd, A.G. (2002). Estimation of spatial variation in risk using matched case–control data. *Biometrical Journal* (to appear).
Kaluzny, S.P., Vega, S.C., Cardoso, T.P. and Shelly, A.A. (1996). *S+Spatial Stats User's Manual*. Seattle: MathSoft.
Kathirgamatamby, N. (1953). Note on the Poisson index of dispersion. *Biometrika*, **40**, 225–8.
Kelly, F.P. and Ripley, B.D. (1976). A note on Strauss' model for clustering. *Biometrika*, **63**, 357–60.
Kelsall, J.E. and Diggle, P.J. (1995a). Kernel estimation of relative risk. *Bernoulli*, **1**, 3–16.
Kelsall, J.E. and Diggle, P.J. (1995b). Nonparametric estimation of spatial variation in relative risk. *Statistics in Medicine*, **14**, 2335–42.
Kelsall, J.E. and Diggle, P.J. (1998). Spatial variation in risk: a nonparametric binary regression approach. *Applied Statistics*, **47**, 559–73.

References

Kendall, M.G. (1970). *Rank Correlation Methods*, 4th edn. London: Griffin.
Kennedy, W.J. and Gentle, J.E. (1980). *Statistical Computing*. New York: Marcel Dekker.
Kershaw, K.A. (1957). The use of cover and frequency in the detection of pattern in plant communities. *Ecology*, **38**, 291–9.
Kershaw, K.A. (1973). *Quantitative and Dynamic Plant Ecology*, 2nd edn. London: Arnold.
Kingman, J.F.C. (1977). Remarks on the spatial distribution of a reproducing population. *Journal of Applied Probability*, **14**, 577–83.
Kulldorff, M. (1997). A spatial scan statistic. *Communications in Statistics: Theory and Methods*, **26**, 1481–96.
Kuldorff, M. (1999). An isotonic spatial scan statistic for geographical disease surveillance. *Journal of the National Institute of Public Health*, **48**, 94–101.
Lawson, A.B (1989). Discussion on cancer near nuclear installations. *Journal of the Royal Statistical Society*, A **152**, 374–5.
Lawson, A.B. (1993). On the analysis of mortality events associated with a prespecified fixed point. *Journal of the Royal Statistical Society*, A **156**, 363–77.
Lewis, P.A.W. and Shedler, G.S. (1979). Simulation of non-homogenous Poisson processes by thinning. *Naval Research Logistics Quarterly*, **26**, 403–13.
Lloyd, M. (1967). Mean crowding. *Journal of Animal Ecology*, **36**, 1–30.
Lotwick H.W. (1981). PhD thesis, University of Bath.
Lotwick, H.W. and Silverman, B.W. (1982). Methods for analysing spatial processes of several types of points. *Journal of the Royal Statistical Society*, B **44**, 406–13.
McCullagh, P. and Nelder, J.A. (1989). *Generalized Linear Models*, 2nd edn. London: Chapman & Hall.
Mannion, D. (1964). Random space-filling in one dimension. *Publications of the Mathematical Institute of the Hungarian Academy of Science*, **9**, 143–53.
Marriott, F.H.C. (1979). Monte Carlo tests: how many simulations? *Applied Statistics*, **28**, 75–7.
Matérn, B. (1960). *Spatial Variation*. Meddelanden fran statens skogsforsningsinstitut, Vol. 49(5). Stockholm: Statens Skogsforsningsinstitut.
Matérn, B. (1971). Doubly stochastic Poisson processes in the plane. In *Statistical Ecology*, Vol. 1, ed. G.P. Patil, E.C. Pielou and W.E. Waters, 195–213. University Park: Pennsylvania State University Press.
Matérn, B. (1986). *Spatial Variation*. New York: Springer.
Matheron, G. (1975). *Random Sets and Integral Geometry*. New York: Wiley.
Maynard-Smith, J. (1974). *Models in Ecology*. London: Cambridge University Press.
Mead, R. (1974). A test for spatial pattern at several scales using data from a grid of contiguous quadrats. *Biometrics*, **30**, 295–307.
Møller, J., Syversveen, A.R. and Waagepetersen, R.P. (1998). Log-Gaussian Cox processes. *Scandinavian Journal of Statistics*, **25**, 451–82.
Møller, J. and Waagepetersen, R.P. (2002). Simulation-based inference for spatial point processes. In *Spatial Statistics and Computational Methods*, ed. J. Møller, 143–99. New York: Springer.
Moore, P.G. (1954). Spacing in plant populations. *Ecology*, **35**, 222–7.
Morisita, M. (1959). Measuring the dispersion of individuals and analysis of the distributional patterns. *Memoirs of the Faculty of Science, Kyushu University Series E* (Biology), **2**, 215–35.
NAG (1977). *Fortran Library Manual*. Oxford: NAG Executive.
Nelder, J.A. and Mead, R. (1965). A simplex method for function minimization. *Computer Journal*, **7**, 308–13.
Neyman, J. (1939). On a new class of contagious distributions, applicable in entomology and bacteriology. *Annals of Mathematical Statistics*, **10**, 35–57.
Neyman, J. and Scott, E.L. (1958). Statistical approach to problems of cosmology (with discussion). *Journal of the Royal Statistical Society*, B **20**, 1–43.

Numata, M. (1961). Forest vegetation in the vicinity of Choshi. Coastal flora and vegetation at Choshi, Chiba Prefecture IV. *Bulletin of Choshi Marine Laboratory, Chiba University*, **3**, 28–48 [in Japanese].

Ogata, Y. and Tanemura, M. (1981). Estimation of interaction potentials of spatial point patterns through the maximum likelihood procedure. *Annals of the Institute of Statistical Mathematics*, B **33**, 315–38.

Ogata, Y. and Tanemura, M. (1984). Likelihood analysis of spatial point patterns. *Journal of the Royal Statistical Society*, B **46**, 496–518.

Ogata, Y. and Tanemura, M. (1986). Likelihood estimation of interaction potentials and external fields of inhomogeneous spatial point patterns. In *Pacific Statistical Congress*, ed. I.S. Francis, B.J.F. Manly and F.C. Lam, 150–4. Amsterdam: Elsevier.

Patil, S.A., Burnham, K.P. and Kovner, J.L. (1979). Non-parametric estimation of plant density by the distance method. *Biometrics*, **35**, 613–22.

Peebles, P.J.E. (1974). The nature of the distribution of galaxies. *Astronomy and Astrophysics*, **32**, 197–202.

Penttinen, A. (1984). *Modelling Interaction in Spatial Point Patterns: Parameter Estimation by the Maximum Likelihood Method*. Jyväskylä Studies in Computer Science, Economics and Statistics, 7. University of Jyväskylä.

Perry, J.N. and Mead, R. (1979). On the power of the index of dispersion test to detect spatial pattern. *Biometrics*, **35**, 613–22.

Persson, O. (1964). Distance methods. *Studia Forestalia Suecica*, **15**, 1–68.

Persson, O. (1971). The robustness of estimating density by distance measurements. In *Statistical Ecology*, Vol. 2, ed. G.P. Patil, E.C. Pielou and W.E. Waters, 175–90. University Park: Pennsylvania State University Press.

Pollard, J.H. (1971). On distance estimators of density in randomly distributed forests. *Biometrics*, **27**, 991–1002.

Preston, C.J. (1977). Spatial birth-and-death processes. *Bulletin of the International Statistical Institute*, **46**(2), 371–91.

Rathbun, S.L. (1996). Estimation of Poisson intensity using partially observed concomitant variables. *Biometrics*, **52**, 226–42.

Ripley, B.D. (1976). The second-order analysis of stationary point processes. *Journal of Applied Probability*, **13**, 255–66.

Ripley, B.D. (1977). Modelling spatial patterns (with discussion). *Journal of the Royal Statistical Society*, B **39**, 172–212.

Ripley, B.D. (1978). Spectral analysis and the analysis of pattern in plant communities. *Journal of Ecology*, **66**, 965–81.

Ripley, B.D. (1979a). Tests of 'randomness' for spatial point patterns. *Journal of the Royal Statistical Society*, B **41**, 368–74.

Ripley, B.D. (1979b). Simulating spatial patterns: dependent samples from a multivariate density. *Applied Statistics*, **28**, 109–12.

Ripley, B.D. (1981). *Spatial Statistics*. New York: Wiley.

Ripley, B.D. (1987). *Stochastic Simulation*. New York: Wiley.

Ripley, B.D. (1988). *Statistical Inference for Spatial Processes*. Cambridge: Cambridge University Press.

Ripley, B.D. and Kelly, F.P. (1977). Markov point processes. *Journal of the London Mathematical Society*, **15**, 188–92.

Ripley, B.D. and Silverman, B.W. (1978). Quick tests for spatial regularity. *Biometrika*, **65**, 641–2.

Rogers, C.A. (1964). *Packing and Covering*. London: Cambridge University Press.

Rowlingson, B.S. and Diggle, P.J. (1993). Splancs: Spatial point pattern analysis code in S-Plus. *Computers in Geosciences*, **19**, 627–55.

References

Särkkä, A. (1993). *Pseudo-likelihood Approach for Pair Potential Estimation of Gibbs Processes*. Jyväskylä Studies in Computer Science, Economics and Statistics, 22. University of Jyväskylä.

Selvin, H.C. (1958). Durkheim's 'suicide' and problems of empirical research. *American Journal of Sociology*, **63**, 607–19.

Silverman, B.W. (1981). Density estimation for univariate and bivariate data. In *Interpreting Multivariate Data*, ed. V. Barnett, 37–53. Chichester: Wiley.

Silverman, B.W. and Brown, T. (1978). Short distances, flat triangles and Poisson limits. *Journal of Applied Probability*, **15**, 815–25.

Skellam, J.G. (1958). On the derivation and applicability of Neyman's Type A distribution. *Biometrika*, **45**, 32–6.

Sprent, P. (1981). *Quick Statistics*. Harmondsworth: Penguin.

Stein, M.L. (1991). A new class of estimators for the reduced second moment measure of point processes. *Biometrika*, **78**, 281–6.

Stiteler, W.M. and Patil, G.P. (1971). Variance to mean ratio and Morisita's index as measures of spatial pattern in ecological populations. In *Statistical Ecology*, Vol. 1, ed. G.P. Patil, E.C. Pielou and W.E. Waters, 423–59. University Park: Pennsylvania State University Press.

Stoyan, D. (1979). Interrupted point processes. *Biometrical Journal*, **21**, 607–10.

Stoyan, D., Kendall, W.S. and Mecke, J. (1995). *Stochastic Geometry and its Applications*, 2nd edn. New York: Wiley.

Stoyan, D. and Stoyan, H. (1994). *Fractals, Random Shapes and Point Fields*. New York: Wiley.

Strauss, D.J. (1975). A model for clustering. *Biometrika*, **62**, 467–75.

Tanemura, M. (1979). On random complete packing by discs. *Annals of the Institute of Statistical Mathematics*, **31**, 351–65.

Tango, T. (1995). A class of tests for detecting 'general' and 'focused' clustering of rare diseases. *Statistics in Medicine*, **14**, 2323–34.

Tango, T. (2000). A test for spatial disease clustering adjusted for multiple testing. *Statistics in Medicine*, **19**, 191–204.

Thomas, M. (1949). A generalization of Poisson's binomial limit for use in ecology. *Biometrika*, **36**, 18–25.

Thompson, H.R. (1956). Distribution of distance to nth nearest neighbour in a population of randomly distributed individuals. *Ecology*, **37**, 391–4.

Townsend, P., Phillimore, P. and Beattie, Q.A. (1988). *Health and Deprivation: Inequalities and the North*. London: Croom Helm.

Upton, G.J.G. and Fingleton, B. (1985). *Spatial Data Analysis by Example, Volume 1: Point Pattern and Quantitative Data*. Chichester: Wiley.

Upton, G.J.G. and Fingleton, B. (1989). *Spatial Data Analysis by Example, Volume 2: Categorical and Directional Data*. Chichester: Wiley.

Van Lieshout, M.N.M. (2000). *Markov Point Processes and Their Applications*. London: Imperial College Press.

Van Lieshout, M.N.M. and Baddeley, A.J. (1996). A nonparametric measure of spatial interaction in point processes. *Statistical Neerlandica*, **50**, 344–61.

Venables, W.N. and Ripley, B.D. (1994). *Modern Applied Statistics with S-Plus*. New York: Springer.

Warren, W.G. (1971). The centre satellite concept as a basis for ecological sampling. In *Statistical Ecology*, Vol. 2, ed. G.P. Patil, E.C. Pielou and W.E. Waters, 87–116. University Park: Pennsylvania State University Press.

Warren, W.G. and Batcheler, C.L. (1979). The density of spatial patterns: robust estimation through distance methods. In *Spatial and Temporal Analysis in Ecology*, ed. R.M. Cormack and J. K. Ord, 240–70. Fairland, MD: International Co-operative Publishing House.

Wichmann, B.A. and Hill, I.D. (1982). Algorithm AS183. An efficient and portable pseudo-random number generator. *Applied Statistics*, **31**, 188–90. (Correction: **33**, 123.)

Williams, J.R., Alexander, F.E., Cartwright, R.A. and McNally, R.J.Q. (2001). Methods for eliciting aetiological clues from geographically clustered cases of disease, with application to leukaemia-lymphoma data. *Journal of the Royal Statistical Society*, A **164**, 49–60.

Woodward, M. (1999). *Epidemiology: Study Design and Data Analysis*. Boca Raton: Chapman & Hall CRL.

Index

amacrine cell data
  Monte Carlo tests 113–14
  spatial point processes 58–60, 109–10
arbitrary point, nearest event **35**
asthma in N Derbyshire 137
asymptotic distribution theory, Monte Carlo tests 10

biological cell *Spatial Point Patterns*
  CSR
    inter-event distances 16
    nearest neighbour distances 19–20
    point-to-nearest-event distances 22–3
    quadrat counts 25
  see also amacrine cell data; brain tissue; cancer;
blurred critical regions 9
brain tissue, pyramidal neurons
  normal **122**, 124–7
  schizophrenia 124–7
bramble cane patterns
  Cox process 97–8
  goodness-of-fit using nearest neighbour distributions 92–100
buffer zone method, edge effects 5

cancers
  childhood leukaemia, N Humberside 131–2
  hamster tumour data, parameter estimation via goodness-of-fit 100–3
  N Liverpool 137–41
Catana's wandering quarter **38**
Chetwynd–Diggle
  statistic D 132
chi-square
  inter-event distances 14
  tests of independence 40–1
childhood asthma, N Derbyshire, point source models 137
Clark–Evans test 18, 20, 93
clique, defined 74

clustering, and heterogeneity, methods in spatial epidemiology 143–4
complete spatial randomness (CSR) 6–7
  distribution theory under CSR 33–5
  inter-event distances 13–14
  Monte Carlo tests 22, 60
  statistical analysis 7–8
  tests 12–13, 31–2
  scale-free statistic 36
contagious distributions 32, 63–4
continuous spatial distribution (CSR) models 63–85
  contagious distributions 63–4
  Cox processes 68–71
  inhomogeneous Poisson processes 67–8
  Markov point processes 74–8
  multivariate models 82–85
    Cox processes 83–5
    formulation 82–3
    marked point processes 82
    Markov point processes 85
    multivariate point processes 82
  other constructions 78–82
    interactions in an inhomogeneous environment 81–2
    lattice-based processes 78–9
    superpositions 80–1
    thinned processes 79–80
  Poisson cluster processes 64–7
  simple inhibition processes 72–4
covariance density, defined 44
Cox processes 68–71, **70**, 83–5
  bramble cane nearest neighbour distributions 97–8
  log-Gaussian 71
  multivariate models 83–5
  thinned processes 79–80

Delaunay triangulation **8**
Dirichlet tesselation **8**–10
  Green–Sibson algorithm 21
  nearest neighbour distances 18–19

disease, area-level studies   128
dispersal of offspring
   simulations of Poisson cluster processes
      87–8
   see also Lansing Woods Michigan, data;
      seedling *SPPs*
distance measurements   33–40
   distribution theory under CSR   33–5
   estimators of intensity   39–40
   tests of CSR   35–9
distance methods of sampling   4, 33–40
distribution functions
   $F(x)$ 46
   $G(y)$ 18, 42, 46
   inter-event distances   28–9
   see also empirical distribution function
      (EDF)

ecological fallacy, defined   128
edge effects
   buffer zone method   5
   sampling   5–6
   toroidal wrapping   5–6
empirical distribution function (EDF)
   examples   61–2
   goodness-of-fit assessment   89
   inter-event distances   13
      plots   **15–16**
   nearest neighbour distances   17–20
epidemiology
   area-level and individual-level studies
      128
   multivariate models   83
   see also point process methods in spatial
      epidemiology
events
   defined   1
   intensity   6, 7, 30, 32
   inter-event distances   13–17

$F(x)$
   defined   46
   estimation   60

Gaussian distribution, $K(t)$-function   87
geostatistics   83
goodness-of-fit
   nearest neighbour distribution   89–90,
      99
   parameter estimation   100–3
Green–Sibson Dirichlet tesselation algorithm
   21

Greig–Smith procedure, scales of pattern
   defect   25
$G(y)$ 18, 42, 46
   defined   46
   estimator   60

hamster tumour data, parameter estimation
   via goodness-of-fit   100–3
heterogeneity, and clustering, methods in
   spatial epidemiology   143–4
homogeneous Poisson process   47–8,
   82–5

independence
   tests   40–1
   univariate processes   48–9
index of dispersion   25–6, 31–2
   power   32
   scales of pattern   25–8
inhibition processes
   K-functions   102
   simple sequential   72–4, **73**
intensity   6, 7, 30, 32
   estimates   32
   estimators   39–40
inter-event distances   13–17
   distribution function   28–9

J-functions
   $J(t)$ 60, 115–16

K-functions
   bootstrapped data   123–4
   case and control   131
   estimating from replicated data,
      non-parametric methods   123–4
   inhibition processes   102
   $K(t)$
      Ripley's estimator   **50**
      second-order processes   49–55
      stationary isotropic process   43–5
      unknown, procedure   88
   $K_{11}(t)$ 49
   $K_{12}(t)$ 48, 98
   $K_{ij}(t)$ 46, 127
   $K_I(t)$ 106
   $K_s(t)$ 88
   parameter estimation   86–8
   pyramidal neurons, brain tissue   **122**
   simulations of Poisson cluster processes
      87–8
kernel estimators   117

Lansing Woods Michigan, data 26–7
  estimation of spatially varying intensity 118–21
  fitting a trend surface 105–6
  sparse sampling 32–3
  T sampling 40
  see also seedling SPPs
lattice-based CSR processes 78–9
least squares estimation, using K-function 86–7
leukaemia, children in N Humberside 131–2
likelihood ratio statistic, Poisson log-linear model 124
likelihood-based methods of model-fitting 104–14
  Monte Carlo tests 110–12
Lotwick–Silverman, $K(t)$, Poisson process 51, 53–5

Markov chain, Monte Carlo algorithm 78
Markov point processes 74–8, 107–14
  likelihood function 74–5
  likelihood interference 107
  Markov of range p 74
  model-fitting using likelihood-based methods 107–14
  more general forms of interaction 78
  multivariate models 85
  pairwise interaction point processes 75–8
    bivariate 85
  Strauss process 75
Markov random fields 4
Mead's procedure
  scales of dependence 27
  scales of pattern 25–8
mean square error (MSE) 116–17
mineral exploration, multivariate models 83
model-fitting using likelihood-based methods 104–14
  inhomogenous Poisson processes 104–6
    fitting trend surface to Lansing Woods data 105–6
  Markov point processes 107–14
    displaced amacrine cells 109–10, 113–14
    fitting pairwise interaction point process to displaced amacrine cells 109–10
    maximum pseudo-likelihood estimation 107–9
    Monte Carlo maximum likelihood estimation 110–12
    non-parametric estimation of a pairwise interaction function 109

model-fitting using summary descriptions 86–103
  goodness-of-fit using nearest neighbour distributions 89–103
    bramble canes 92–100
    examples 90–100
    parameter estimation 100
    analysis of hamster tumour data 100–3
    redwood seedlings 90–2
  parameter estimation using K-function 86–8
    least squares estimation 86–7
    procedure when $K(t)$ is unknown 88
    simulations of Poisson cluster processes 87–8
Monte Carlo algorithm, Markov chain 78
Monte Carlo tests 9
  amacrine cell data 113–14
  asymptotic distribution theory 10
  blurred critical regions **10**
  complete spatial randomness (CSR) 22, 60
  maximum likelihood estimation 110–12
  significance levels 89
multivariate models 82–85

$N(dx)$ process 79
nearest event, arbitrary point **35**
nearest neighbour distances 17–20
nearest neighbour distribution
  analysis, goodness-of-fit 89–90, 99
  estimation 60–2
  functions 80, **81**
neighbours, defined 74
non-parametric methods 115–27
  analysing replicated spatial point patterns 121–7
    between-group comparisons in designed experiments 124–7
    estimating K-function from replicated data 123–4
    parametric vs non-parametric methods 127
  estimation of a spatially varying intensity 116–21
    Lansing Woods data 118–21
$N_j(S)$ 45

pairwise interaction point processes 75–8
  displaced amacrine cells 109–10
  inhibitory, thinning **80**
  non-parametric estimation 109
parameter estimation, using K-function 86–8

158 Index

parametric vs non-parametric methods, analysing replicated spatial point patterns   127
plant distribution *see* bramble; Lansing Woods Michigan, data; seedling *SPPs*
plotless sampling techniques   33–40
    see also distance methods
point process methods in spatial epidemiology   128–44
    cancers in N Liverpool   137–41
    disentangling heterogeneity and clustering   143–4
    point source models   134–7
        childhood asthma in N Derbyshire, England   137
        elevation of risk, directional model   **136**
    spatial clustering   130–3
        N Humberside childhood leukaemia data   131–2
        other tests   132–3
    spatial variation in risk   133–4
    stratification and matching   141–3
point-to-nearest-event distances   21–3
Poisson distributions
    contagious   63–4
    log-linear model, likelihood ratio statistic   124
    quadrat counts   24
Poisson processes   18, 28, 42
    cluster   64–7
        simulations, K-function, model-fitting   87–8
    examples   56–8
    homogeneous   47–8, 82–5
    inhomogeneous   55, 67–8, 81–2, 104–6
        quadratic trend surface model   105, **106**
    $K(t)$
        Chetwynd–Diggle   51–5
        Lotwick–Silverman   51, 53–5
        superposition   81
    linked pairs bivariate process   84
    multivariate Cox processes   83–5
    point process models   63–85
    and Poisson cluster process   81
    postulates   47
    simulation   53
preliminary testing   12–29
    inter-event distances   13–18
    nearest neighbour distances   18–20
    point-to-nearest-event distances   21–3
    quadrat counts   23–5
    recommendations   28–9

scales of pattern   25–8
tests of CSR   12–13
$p_n(A)$, quadrat count distribution   45
pyramidal neurons, brain tissue
    normal   **122**
    in schizophrenia   124–7

quadrat counts   23–5, 29
    contagious distributions   32, 63–4
    distribution $p_n(A)$ 45
    Poisson distribution   24
    scales of pattern   25–8
    sparse sampling
        intensity   7, 30, 32
        patterns   31–3
quadrat sampling   3

random labelling, univariate processes   48–9
redwood seedlings *see* seedling *SPPs*
references   144–53
replicated spatial point patterns, analysis   121–7
retinal amacrine cells *see* amacrine cell data
Ripley's asymptotic approximation   51
Ripley's estimator, $K(t)$ **50**
risk, spatial variation   133–4

sampling   3–5
    Catana's wandering quarter   **38**
    distance methods   4
    edge effects   5–6
    partitioning   4
    replicated   4–5
    sparse sampling   30–41
        intensity   7, 30, 32
        quadrats   3
    variance-to-mean ratio   25–6
scales of dependence   27–8
scales of pattern   25–8
schizophrenia, brain tissue, pyramidal neurons   **122**, 124–7
second-order properties, estimation   49–58
    inhomogeneous Poisson processes   55
    multivariate   55–6
    univariate   49–55
seedling *SPPs*
    calculating density of mature parent trees   91, **92**
    CSR   15–16
    inter-event distances   15–16
    nearest neighbour distances   19–20
        model-fitting   90–2
    point-to-nearest-event distances   22–3

Poisson process, examples 57–8, **91**
  quadrat counts 24–5
  see also Lansing Woods Michigan, data
simple sequential inhibition processes 72–4, **73**
sparsely sampled patterns 30–41
  intensity 7, 30, 32
  quadrat counts 31–3
  recommendations 28–9
  tests of independence 40–1
spatial clustering 130–3
spatial point patterns
  complete spatial randomness (CSR) 6–7
  defined 1–3
  multivariate 2–3
  preliminary testing 12–29
  replicated, analysis 121–7
  software 10–11
spatial point processes 42–62
  amacrine cell data 58–60
  defined 42
  estimation of nearest neighbour distributions 60–2
  estimation of second-order properties 49–58
  examples 61–2
  first-order processes 43
  higher-order moments and nearest neighbour distributions 46
  homogeneous Poisson process 47–8, 82–5
  independence and random labelling 48–9
  second-order processes 43–6

spatial variation in risk 133–4
  point source models 134–6
  stratification 143
Splancs software 11, 50
SPPs see spatial point patterns
stationarity assumption, defined 42
stationary processes
  $K(t)$ 43
  reweighted 43–5
statistical analysis
  objectives 7–8
  recommendations 28–9
  sparsely sampled patterns 30–41
stochastic models, defined 2
stratification and matching 141–3
  benefits 143
  individually matched case-control designs 141–3
  stratified case-control designs 141
Strauss process, pairwise interaction point processes 75–8, 103

T-square sampling **35**, 37
tessellations, Dirichlet 8–10
thinned processes 79–80
toroidal wrapping 5–6
trees *see* Lansing Woods Michigan, data

variance-to-mean ratio (index of dispersion) 25–6, 31–2
  lattice patterns 32
Voronoi tesselation 8–10